Ethical Issues in Forensic
Psychiatry

Ethical Issues in Forensic Psychiatry

Minimizing Harm

By

Robert L. Sadoff, MD
University of Pennsylvania, Philadelphia, USA

with contributions from

John A. Baird, MD
Royal College of Psychiatrists, Leverndale Hospital, Glasgow, UK

Solange Margery Bertoglia, MD
Thomas Jefferson University Hospital, Philadelphia, USA

Emanuele Valenti, MBe, PhD
European University of Madrid, Madrid, Spain

Donna L. Vanderpool, MBA, JD
Professional Risk Management Services, Inc., Arlington, USA

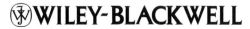

WILEY-BLACKWELL

A John Wiley & Sons, Ltd., Publication

This edition first published 2011 © 2011 by John Wiley & Sons Ltd

Wiley-Blackwell is an imprint of John Wiley & Sons, formed by the merger of Wiley's global Scientific, Technical and Medical business with Blackwell Publishing.

Registered office: John Wiley & Sons Ltd, The Atrium, Southern Gate, Chichester, West Sussex, PO19 8SQ, UK

Editorial offices: 9600 Garsington Road, Oxford, OX4 2DQ, UK
111 River Street, Hoboken, NJ 07030-5774, USA

For details of our global editorial offices, for customer services and for information about how to apply for permission to reuse the copyright material in this book please see our website at www.wiley.com/wiley-blackwell.

Library of Congress Cataloging-in-Publication Data
Sadoff, Robert L., 1936-
  Ethical issues in forensic psychiatry : minimizing harm / by Robert L. Sadoff ; with contributions from John A. Baird ... [et al.].
    p. cm.
  Includes bibliographical references and index.
  ISBN 978-0-470-67013-2 (cloth : alk. paper)   1.   Forensic psychiatry–Moral and ethical aspects.
I. Baird, John A.   II.   Title.
  [DNLM: 1.   Forensic Psychiatry–ethics. W 740 S126e 2011]
  RA1151.S227 2011
  614'.15–dc22

                                                                                          2010023321

A catalogue record for this book is available from the British Library

This book is published in the following electronic formats: eBook [9780470971871]; Wiley Online Library [9780470971888]

Set in 10.5/12.5 Times Roman by Laserwords Private Limited, Chennai, India
Printed in Singapore by Ho Printing Singapore Pte Ltd

1   2011

"The Highest Form of Wisdom is Kindness"
The Talmud

Contents

About the Authors

Robert L. Sadoff, MD

Dr. Sadoff is currently Clinical Professor of Forensic Psychiatry and Director of the Forensic Psychiatry Fellowship at the University of Pennsylvania School of Medicine. Dr. Sadoff received his MD in 1959 from the University of Minnesota School of Medicine and completed his residency in psychiatry in 1963 at UCLA Neuropsychiatric Institute, from which he received a master of science degree in psychiatry. He also attended Temple University School of Law and has taught legal medicine courses at Temple University Law School and at the Villanova University School of Law. He is board certified in psychiatry, forensic psychiatry, and legal medicine, and has added qualifications in forensic psychiatry with the American Board of Psychiatry and Neurology.

Dr. Sadoff is the author of over 90 articles in medical and legal journals and more than 30 chapters in books by other authors, and has authored, edited, or co-authored eight books, including *Forensic Psychiatry: A Practical Guide for Lawyers and Psychiatrists, Psychiatric Malpractice: Cases and Comments for Clinicians*, with Robert I. Simon, MD, *Mental Health Experts: Roles and Qualifications for Court* and *Crime and Mental Illness* with Frank Dattilio, PhD. He has numerous editorial appointments with peer reviewed journals. He has served as President of the American Academy of Psychiatry and the Law, and President of the American Board of Forensic Psychiatry. In addition, he is a Distinguished Life Fellow of the American Psychiatric Association, a Fellow of the American College of Legal Medicine, and a Fellow of the American Academy of Forensic Sciences, as well as a Fellow of the American College of Psychiatrists and The College of Physicians of Philadelphia, for which he serves on the board of trustees.

Dr. Sadoff is the recipient of a number of national and international awards, including the very prestigious Isaac Ray Award from the American Psychiatric Association, the Philippe Pinel Award given by the International Academy of

Law and Mental Health, the Lifetime Achievement Award from the Philadelphia Psychiatric Society, and the Earl Bond Award and the Dean's Special Award from the University of Pennsylvania. In addition, he has been the recipient of the Manfred S. Guttmacher Award from the American Psychiatric Association, and the recipient of the Nathaniel Winkelman Award from the Philadelphia Psychiatric Center. He has also been named repeatedly in the list of *Best Doctors in America* and in *Who's Who in America* and *Who's Who in the World*.

Dr. Sadoff has examined over 10 000 individuals charged with crimes during the past 40 years, and has testified for both the prosecution and defense in criminal cases and for the plaintiff and defense in civil cases in approximately 20 states and several federal jurisdictions. He has served as a consultant to the Norristown State Hospital, the Trenton Psychiatric Hospital, the Harrisburg State Hospital and the Forensic Psychiatric Hospital of New Jersey, as well as the Philadelphia prison system. Dr. Sadoff has been licensed to practice medicine in five states, including Pennsylvania, New York, California, Minnesota, and New Jersey (currently inactive). He has also lectured in nearly all of the states in the United States and in 12 countries worldwide.

John A. Baird, MD, FRCPsych DCH

Dr. John Baird has worked as a forensic psychiatrist in Scotland for over 30 years. He has in the past been a member of the Parole Board for Scotland, and is currently a member of the Parole Board for England and Wales and the Mental Health Tribunal for Scotland. He is an elected officer of the Executive Committee of the Forensic Faculty of the Royal College of Psychiatrists, having served in the past as Secretary and currently serving as Finance Officer. He has served as a member of the Ethics Committee of the Royal College of Psychiatrists. His MD thesis was a study of psychiatric aspects of imprisonment in Scotland.

Solange Margery Bertoglia, MD
Assistant Professor of Psychiatry, Jefferson Hospital

Dr. Solange Margery Bertoglia was born and raised in Costa Rica by her Chilean immigrant parents and older brothers. She received her MD degree from the Universidad de Costa Rica, before emigrating to the United States. Dr. Margery completed her psychiatry residency training at Temple University Hospital in Philadelphia. During her residency, she served as a liaison between patients from a primarily Latino community and the Department of Psychiatry. Subsequently, she completed her forensic psychiatry fellowship training at Saint Vincent's Catholic Medical Center in New York City. Dr. Margery has researched and made national and local presentations on a variety of forensic issues, including: sex offenders, competency to stand trial, insanity defense, race and ethnicity, and homicide by adolescents. Dr. Margery is currently on the faculty of Thomas Jefferson University in Philadelphia where she is actively involved in the teaching and development of the forensic psychiatry curriculum.

Emanuele Valenti, PhD
Professor of Bioethics and Medical Humanities at Universidad Europea de Madrid, Spain.

Emanuele Valenti holds a Ph.D. from the Universidad Complutense de Madrid, Spain, Department of Preventive Medicine, Public Health, and History of Science under the direction of bioethicist Dr. Diego Gracia. He earned a B.A. in Philosophy from the Universitá degli Studi di Milano, Italy. In Philadelphia, US, he has been research scholar at the Centre for Bioethics, University of Pennsylvania, collaborating in the ScattergoodEthics Program under the direction of Dr. Arthur Caplan. As visiting scholar, Dr. Valenti has participated in An Observational Descriptive Study of IRB Practices project research under the direction of Dr. Charles Lidz in the Center for Mental Health Services Research at the Worcester State Hospital, University of Massachusetts. He has worked as researcher in the Center for Bioethics and Health Governance at the Hospital Policlinico di Milano, Italy, where he has developed a program to promote a good practice of informed consent. His primary research focuses on coercive measures in mental health, and the assessment of the impact of coercion in the decision making capacity of the patient. He is currently working on the reform and harmonization of the European mental health system.

Donna L. Vanderpool, MBA, JD
Services Assistant Vice President, Risk Management
Professional Risk Management Services, Inc.

Ms. Vanderpool, a healthcare attorney, is the Assistant Vice President of Risk Management at PRMS, a company that manages all aspects of a professional liability insurance program for psychiatrists and other mental health professionals. In addition to assisting the Vice President with the development and implementation of risk management services, she staffs the Risk Management Consultation Service Helpline, giving telephone advice on all types of psychiatric risk management issues, and contributes to PRMS' publications and seminars. She is a frequent speaker for a variety of organizations throughout the nation on psychiatric risk management topics and has had risk management articles published in legal and psychiatric journals. Ms. Vanderpool has also developed a particular interest and expertise in the area of forensic liability. Ms. Vanderpool's professional background includes practicing criminal defense, teaching business and legal courses, and managing a general surgical practice. Ms. Vanderpool received her undergraduate degree from James Madison University and her MBA and JD from George Mason University.

Luis Fernando Barrios Flores, JD
Dr. Barrios graduated in Law from the University of Salamanca (Spain) and is a Juridical Doctor at the University of Alicante (Spain). He has worked in Spanish

penitentiary institutions for over 30 years. His JD thesis was a study on the Juridical Statute of the Patient.

Dr. Barrios is the author of 6 books, over 50 articles published in medical and legal journals, and has contributed 18 chapters to books by other authors.

He has intervened, as a member of the legal expert panel, in the following studies: EUNOMIA (European Evaluation of Coercion in Psychiatry and Harmonisation of Best Clinical Practice, within the Fifth Framework Programme of Research of the European Commission, completed in 2005), EUPRIS (Mentally ill or disordered persons in European prison systems—Needs, Programmes and Outcome, European Commission, completed in 2007), DEMoB.inc (Development of a European Measure of Best Practice for People with Long Term Mental Illness in Institutional Care, European Commission, completed in 2010).

Dr. Barrios is a member of the Geneva International Academic Network on Mental Health, Human Rights and Legislation of the World Health Organization (WHO), and he has collaborated with the Pan American Health Organization (OPS). He is a co-author of the report: "Fundamental Freedoms, Basic Rights and Care for the Mentally Ill" (Council of Europe, 2009–10).

Preface

Isaac Ray

This book is dedicated to the memory of Isaac Ray, the great nineteenth century American psychiatrist who became the father of American forensic psychiatry following the publication of his seminal book, *A Treatise on the Medical Jurisprudence of Insanity*, published initially in Boston, in 1838 [1]. Dr. Ray was instrumental in advocating for the rights of the mentally ill, for protection of those who were less able to protect themselves, and advocated for reforms that are still needed today.

The forensic psychiatric historian, Dr. Jacques Quen, in a paper entitled, "Isaac Ray: Have We Learned His Lessons?" [2] cites Overholser and Weihofen, who summarized Isaac Ray's philosophy as "doing as little harm to the mentally ill as possible." The authors quote Ray as stating, "In the first place, the law should put no hindrance in the way of the prompt use of those instrumentalities which are regarded as most effectual in promoting the comfort and restoration of the patient. Secondly, it should spare all unnecessary exposure of private troubles, and all unnecessary conflict with popular prejudices. Thirdly, it should protect individuals from wrongful imprisonment" [3].

Although Ray was most concerned about commitment of the mentally ill and the manner in which the mentally ill were treated in judicial decisions in court cases, his concern about doing little or no harm is the basic theme of this book, in which I hope to illustrate means by which we may limit or minimize the inherent harm in the practice of forensic psychiatry.

Primum Non Nocere

The concept of *primum non nocere*—first, do no harm—is the basis for ethical medical practice and treatment in psychiatry. However, it cannot, and does not, apply to forensic cases where there is no doctor-patient relationship and the forensic psychiatrist may indeed cause harm to the examinee. Consider, for example, the psychiatrist hired by the prosecution in a capital murder case. His or her assessment of the defendant may lead to a verdict of guilty and subsequent death penalty. Consider also the role of the treating psychiatrist on death row, treating a psychotic prisoner who has deteriorated and requires medication and further therapy in order to improve to the point where he or she may be competent to be executed. Consider also the plaintiff in a civil matter who has been emotionally harmed as well as physically damaged in an accident or incident at work. Consider the forensic psychiatrist working for the defense in that case who may minimize the damage or find no significant mental illness caused by the accident in question.

Forensic psychiatrists work in three major areas in assessment of individuals in civil or criminal cases. First, they are involved in examining the defendant in a criminal case, or the plaintiff in a civil matter. Secondly, they are responsible for writing a report to the court or to an attorney regarding their findings, which would include not only the psychiatric examination, but also the review of extensive records and interviewing collaborative individuals, when necessary. Third, they may be required to testify at deposition and/or at trial. Harm may come to the individual examined at any or all of the three levels of work: examination, report writing, and/or testimony.

Personal Concerns

I have been practicing psychiatry for over 45 years, 25 years of which have been exclusively in forensic work. During the past many years I have seen over 12 000 individuals, either in civil or criminal cases, in a variety of different circumstances. I have worked for both defense and prosecution in over 10 000 criminal cases, and either for the defendant or the plaintiff in over 2000 civil cases. In addition, I have been asked by judges to evaluate and assess individuals in both criminal and civil matters and have worked in a number of administrative cases involving patients' rights, competency, and other forensic psychiatric issues.

I have been concerned about the manner in which individuals, families, or groups of people have been assessed and the conclusions that have been drawn depending on the needs of the attorney. I have seen testimony that has been slanted, unscientific, and based on inadequate evidence or which is contrary to the facts proven. Perhaps, adversaries of mine in specific cases may have felt the same about my assessments or my testimony. Nevertheless, it is an issue that forensic psychiatrists, attorneys, judges, and other concerned citizens need to address as the practice of forensic psychiatry has grown and proliferated over the past several decades. We now have formal accredited training programs in forensic psychiatry. We have board certification that originated with the American Board of Forensic Psychiatry and which culminated in the acceptance of forensic psychiatry as a subspecialty of psychiatry by the American Board of Psychiatry and Neurology. We have recertification of these boards in forensic psychiatry to insure high quality of professional behavior.

I have been struck with the manner in which colleagues and adversaries have approached their professional responsibilities. I have witnessed destructive and biased attitudes toward various criminal defendants and plaintiffs in civil cases that are unnecessary and harmful. I have witnessed psychiatrists becoming adversarial in order "to win" cases. I have seen professional psychiatrists testify to speculative rather than evidence-based or scientific matters. And I have also seen our colleagues testify on matters for which they have no expertise and very little experience. One psychiatrist even admitted that he did not know the legal criteria for assessing competency in a particular criminal case. Nevertheless, he speculated on the issue based on his medical diagnosis rather than applying the medical observations to the legal standards.

Changes in Psychiatry

Psychiatry is a changing and evolving specialty of medicine. When I began my career in 1960, the emphasis was on psychodynamics, and Freud was still a very prominent influence in the training programs. During the past five decades, we have seen a major shift from psychoanalytic concepts to cognitive behavioral matters in psychotherapy and to chemical imbalance in our diagnoses, and the use of various medications to treat major mental illnesses. Psychopharmacology has become a major subspecialty of psychiatry. In addition, we have developed various techniques to diagnose brain problems, including MRI, PET scan, and CAT scans. Neuropsychological testing has been shown to be effective in the diagnosis of functional organic conditions that may not be revealed on more grossly sensitive tests that pick up only structural organic damage.

We have brought the newer scientific psychiatry into the courtroom when testifying for individuals revealing significant mental illness or brain damage that affected behavior in criminal or civil cases. As a result of the transitions within psychiatry, the law has made further demands on our scientific acumen by such cases as Daubert [4] and Kumho [5], demanding scientific-based testimony rather than speculative "junk science." The judge has become the gatekeeper for various types of testimony that may be harmful to an individual as it reveals prejudice or bias rather than scientific methods.

Bias in Forensic Psychiatry

Several decades ago, one of the early leaders in forensic psychiatry, Bernard Diamond, pointed out, in his historic paper on "The Fallacy of the Impartial Expert" [6], that all of us have our biases that need to be considered in forensic cases.

The major ethical prohibition in medicine has been *primum non nocere*—first, do no harm. Paul Appelbaum [7] and others have shown that forensic psychiatrists have a different ethical standard when conducting assessments, or even in testimony, because the nature of our work cannot guarantee that no harm is done to the individual. Rather, he has developed concepts of respecting the integrity of the evaluee (the defendant in a criminal case, or the plaintiff in a civil case), and considering beneficence or non-maleficence. Others have debated with Appelbaum on these concepts, most notably Alan Stone [8] pointing out glaring differences. This book will attempt to present the major issues that arise for forensic psychiatrists practicing in this very complex and controversial field where harm may occur.

Medicine in General

It is well known that in medicine generally, physicians attempt to treat or cure illnesses by utilizing treatments that may be harmful to patients. However, physicians are clearly aware that in many cases, in order to help their patients, they must first cause pain either through surgery, through various medications or chemotherapy, or other procedures. Even in psychiatry, we have learned that various medications given to improve psychotic conditions may cause harmful side effects such as tardive dyskinesia. We have recently found that some antidepressants may also lead to diabetic conditions. Clearly, electroshock treatment which has been helpful for severe depression has caused many patients fear, anxiety, and harm. We have seen the effects of lobotomy on various patients who were not amenable to treatment by other methods, such as psychotherapy, medication, or even electroshock treatment. All of this is performed in order to help our patients who depend upon us for scientific and accurate information and effective therapy.

Benjamin Rush is considered the father of American psychiatry, and his portrait appears on the seal of the American Psychiatric Association. It should be noted that Benjamin Rush, in all his greatness as a physician and the author of one of the earliest textbooks on psychiatry in America, entitled, *Medical Inquiries and Observations Upon the Diseases of the Mind* [9], used leeches for bloodletting as a means of treating his patients. It is well known that some patients did not do well from such harmful treatments. We learn as we go, and sometimes we have learned that the treatment that was once thought to be helpful and successful was not scientifically based and proved to be harmful.

We have mentioned surgery as a means of helping others that may be harmful. The surgery may result in a painful after-effect, but pain is not necessarily harmful, and we must consider harmful as having long-term side effects. The short-term downside from surgery that leads to long-term cure or improvement is certainly worth the discomfort. When I speak of harm, I am talking about long-term harm that can be either avoided or minimized through careful planning and application of ethical principles outlined by the American Academy of Psychiatry and the Law [10]. However, even following these principles may not eliminate or minimize harm that is inherent in the system.

I am not advocating that the harm can be totally eliminated, because I know that is impossible in the adversarial system in which forensic psychiatrists work. However, there are means by which harm may be minimized if care is taken during the assessment, the report writing, and the testimony phase of the proceedings.

This book will analyze the ethical issues affecting forensic psychiatric practice, especially those promulgated by the American Academy of Psychiatry and the

Law. Within those guidelines, we will look at individual bias, vulnerability of the examinee, and potential harm to the mental health professional. The book will discuss each of the procedures of the forensic expert separately with respect to minimizing harm.

The scope of forensic psychiatry will be developed from the standpoint of administrative, civil, and criminal cases. The practical issues involved in conducting forensic psychiatric assessments under various conditions will be presented as will special considerations, such as bias, minimizing harm, developing a therapeutic approach, and elaborating on various vulnerable individuals who are frequently examined in forensic cases. These include juveniles, mentally retarded, autistic, sexual assault victims, the elderly, the organically damaged, the psychotic, and the mentally disabled prisoners. The ethical issues in conducting forensic psychiatric examinations and presenting psychiatric testimony in court will also be examined and discussed. Cases illustrating the difficulties involved will punctuate the presentation. Harm may also come to the non-vulnerable defendant or plaintiff in legal cases. We need to minimize the harm that comes to these individuals as well whenever possible. Selecting the vulnerable populations does not imply that we are not concerned about the general populations as well. There are those individuals, primarily in civil cases, who are the victims of harassment, discrimination, and prejudice. These are individuals who may not have specific diagnostic entities that place them in the vulnerable categories. However, they may develop psychiatric syndromes or illnesses as a result of the alleged harassment, discrimination or bias. We also see individuals who are victims of accidents with physical and mental injuries, but who do not have a predisposing illness or psychiatric syndrome.

In criminal cases, we may be asked to examine victims of crime who are not in the vulnerable categories. These are people who may have been shot during a robbery or a kidnapping and may require psychiatric assessment as a result of the injuries sustained in the criminal case.

In administrative matters, we may be asked to evaluate professionals who have been accused of negligence in their work or we may need to assess competency of individuals facing administrative matters. In all of these cases, we need to be careful in our assessment, report writing, and testimony in order to minimize harm.

Any ethical issue pertaining to vulnerable populations applies to all individuals seen in forensic mental health matters. The system has inherent difficulties that may bring harm to those involved that we may be able to mitigate whenever possible. There are situations in which harm will occur to those who have transgressed, and that is a justifiable harm or punishment. However, we are more concerned about innocent people who may be victimized even more because of the legal situation in which they are involved. The very act of filing a lawsuit, with all its ramifications and consequences, affects both plaintiffs and defendants. We must do all we can to minimize harm to all populations, but the vulnerable ones listed above will be stressed since they represent individuals who are most likely to be harmed in the legal system if special care is not taken by the forensic psychiatrist to minimize such harm.

The original manuscript for this book did not include the perspective from Europe and the United Kingdom. Reviewers recommended that we include ethical issues in forensic psychiatry from a more global perspective than just from the United States.

Dr. John Baird, a forensic psychiatrist from Scotland who has had experience in working in the United Kingdom, comments on the differences between the practice of forensic psychiatry in the United Kingdom and the United States. His presentation is from a more systemic view, utilizing different organizations that monitor the practice of forensic psychiatry. In both the United Kingdom and Europe, individual forensic psychiatry appears to be secondary to the institutional application of principles to the mentally disabled within the legal system.

Both Dr. Baird and Dr. Valenti, a forensic psychiatrist and ethicist, present the changes that have occurred in both systems that promote the welfare of the individual involved in the legal system. Dr. Baird focuses on minimizing the harm from the perspective of the forensic psychiatrist and Dr. Valenti on human rights for this same population.

Dr. Valenti presents the very complicated system in the European Union that comprises a number of different countries and cultures and legal systems that have attempted to unify their ethics as regards the mentally ill within the judicial system. Dr. Valenti does not focus particularly on minimizing harm, but does relate the newer ethical principles that affect the mentally ill within the court system in the European Union. He points out that the reforms that have occurred in the last several years have helped the human rights of such people and thus harm to them is minimized. Ideally, an attempt is sought to unify the variety of systems in order to promote human rights and thus minimize harm.

The theme of this book is to minimize the harm inherent in forensic psychiatric practice. Clearly, the intent is to minimize the harm to plaintiffs or defendants, but also to the expert witness as well. Donna Vanderpool, an attorney and risk manager, provides comprehensive coverage of potential liability to expert witnesses, especially those in medical malpractice cases. She points out the inconsistencies of a number of Appellate Court holdings and illustrates the complexity of the emerging liability cases against expert witnesses.

Her intent is to educate expert witnesses to prevent damage or harm to themselves in the course of their work in conducting forensic examinations, writing reports, and testifying in court. As she points out, the harm that may come to a defendant or plaintiff could result in retaliation against the expert for causing such harm. She demonstrates the areas of duty the expert has to the examinee and the areas of liability that may exist for the expert professional. Finally, she presents important guidelines and recommendations for the expert in order to prevent or minimize harm.

The motivation to write this book was the presentation of the Isaac Ray Award given by the American Psychiatric Association in 2006, which required my preparing lectures on important issues in forensic psychiatry. Thus, I decided that the important message for the Isaac Ray Lectures should be a reiteration of Ray's concerns about minimizing harm to vulnerable mentally ill patients and applying his recommendations to the forensic psychiatric profession.

In summary, the purpose of this book is to illustrate the ethical and practical issues that affect forensic psychiatric practice. The question is not what we do, but how we do it, and under what standards, ethical guidelines, and personal values that contribute to the total picture. It is hoped that by such presentation and discussion, vast improvements in the manner in which forensic psychiatry is practiced will occur, resulting in less harm to the examinee and greater credibility to the examiner and our role within the judicial system. Despite the fact that we cannot always adhere to the doctrine of *primum non nocere*, we can minimize the harm caused inherently by the adversarial system in which we participate.

References

1. Ray, I. (1838) *Treatise on the Medical Jurisprudence of Insanity.* Little Brown, Boston.
2. Quen, J.M. (1974) Isaac Ray: have we learned his lessons? Read at the Butler Hospital Isaac Ray Symposium on Human Rights, The Law, and Psychiatric Treatment, May 24, 1974, Providence, Rhode Island.
3. Overholser, W. and Weihofen, H. (1946) Commitment of the mentally ill. *The American Journal of Psychiatry*, **102**, 758–69.
4. *Daubert v. Merrell Dow Pharmaceuticals, Inc.*, 509U.S. 579,113S Ct. 2786, 125L.Ed.2d 469 (1993).
5. *Kumho Tire Company, Ltd. v. Carmichael*, 526U.S. 137,119S Ct. 1167, 143L.Ed.2d 238 (1999).
6. Diamond, B. (1959) The fallacy of the impartial expert. *Archives of Criminal Psychodynamics*, **3**, 221–2.
7. Appelbaum, P.S. (1997) A theory of ethics for forensic psychiatry. *Journal of the American Academy of Psychiatry and the Law*, **25**, 233–47.
8. Stone, A.A. (1984) The ethical boundaries of forensic psychiatry: a view from the ivory tower. *Bulletin of the American Academy of Psychiatry and the Law*, **12**, 209–19.
9. Rush, B. (1812) *Medical Inquiries and Observations Upon the Diseases of the Mind.* Kimber and Richardson, Philadelphia.
10. American Academy of Psychiatry and The Law (2005) *Ethics Guidelines for the Practice of Forensic Psychiatry*. Adopted May 2005. Bloomfield, CT.

Acknowledgments

There are so many people I wish to thank for their creative ideas, their emotional and physical support, and for their commitment and devotion to the preparation of this book. First, I thank my parents for instilling in me a sense of responsibility for those less fortunate and for those for whom we care in medicine. Both my mother and father were graduate pharmacists who took special care in the preparation of medications for patients they served. Both also had an idealistic, ethical view of their role in caring for others.

Next, I thank the Isaac Ray Committee of the American Psychiatric Association for the honor of receiving the Isaac Ray Award in 2006, prompting me to write this book in honor of Isaac Ray. It was my dear friend, Dr. Kenneth Weiss, forensic psychiatrist and psychiatric historian, who led me to the writings of Isaac Ray on minimizing harm to the vulnerable mentally ill in our hospitals. I also wish to thank Dr. Marla Isaacs, forensic psychologist, whose sensitivity in examining a vulnerable child in a very difficult domestic relations case stimulated my thinking about minimizing the harm in the work we do in forensic psychiatry.

I am especially grateful to my two original mentors in forensic psychiatry, Melvin S. Heller, MD, whose enthusiasm and ebullience heightened my interest in this very challenging field, and his colleague at Temple University, the late Professor Samuel Polsky, whose brilliance in the field was matched only by his expansive teaching of courses in law and mental health. I thank my dear friend, Professor Michael Perlin, of the New York Law School, with whom I have worked for over 35 years in many capacities and who has always instilled in me a concern and care for the mentally ill and the mentally disabled. He has fought for their welfare through his work as a public defender in Trenton, New Jersey, as the mental health advocate for New Jersey and through his extremely prolific writing on the legal issues affecting the mentally disabled.

I want to thank all of my teachers and all of my students from whom I have learned more, I suspect, than what I taught them. I am also grateful to my many colleagues in forensic psychiatry, and especially those active in the American

Academy of Psychiatry and the Law whose work I have quoted in this book and whose thinking and creative ideas have stimulated the concepts presented herein. Toward that end, I am especially grateful to Drs. Paul Appelbaum, Richard Ciccone, Thomas Gutheil, Jonas Rappeport, Robert Simon, Robert Weinstock, and Robert Wettstein for their prolific writing and special concerns for ethics in forensic psychiatry and for the welfare of those we serve.

The concept that I present in these pages would not be complete without the addition of Donna Vanderpool's chapter. She is an attorney working in risk management who has given us the legal perspective of forensic psychiatric practice that may be harmful to the practitioner. I am most grateful for her significant contribution to this book.

The early reviewers of the manuscript suggested that I include a European perspective on ethical issues in forensic psychiatry. I am most grateful to Dr. Emanuele Valenti, MBe, PhD, who has contributed a significant chapter on the European perspective and to Dr John Baird for his chapter on forensic psychiatry in the United Kingdom. John Baird, from Scotland, has been a regular speaker at our Seminar in Forensic Psychiatry at the University of Pennsylvania. Finally, I thank my colleague and friend, a regular participant in our Seminar in Forensic Psychiatry at the University, Dr. Solange Margery Bertoglia, for contributing a chapter on immigrants as a vulnerable population. Dr. Margery, who hails from Costa Rica, has experienced the view of the immigrant as well as worked with immigrants within the forensic field. I am very grateful to Solange for her important contribution to this book.

There were a number of references and citations that I was not able to find, but with the help of attorney Tina L. Mazza Ralls, Esquire, I could complete the citations and references. I am grateful to Ms. Ralls for her scholarship and her expertise in the law that is so essential to the accuracy of these references. My dear friend and colleague and co-author of other books on forensic mental health, Dr. Frank Dattilio, clinical and forensic psychologist, reviewed a number of chapters and helped clarify ethical issues relating to forensic psychology. For that I am most grateful.

I am especially indebted to my secretary, Ruth Borock, for her devotion, dedication, and commitment to the arduous task of typing, retyping, and re-editing the chapters of this book.

I am also grateful to Joan Marsh, Fiona Woods and Jessminder Kaur at Wiley-Blackwell and Sangeetha Parthasarthy at Laserwords, India for all their hard work in seeing this project to fruition.

Finally, I am grateful to my dear family who have endured time away from me so that I may finish this manuscript, which took about two years to write. My wife, Joan, has always been the greatest support to me throughout my work in psychiatry and forensic psychiatry and to this day, from an ethical standpoint, she remains my moral compass.

Introduction

Robert L. Sadoff

Medicine is the profession that involves the treatment of illness and research in preventing and treating illnesses. Psychiatry is the specialty of medicine that treats mental and emotional illnesses, organic brain syndromes, and physical illness with emotional manifestations. Forensic psychiatry is the subspecialty of psychiatry that deals with people who are involved in legal matters, either criminal or civil. Treatment psychiatry (sometimes erroneously referred to as clinical psychiatry, since forensic psychiatry is also clinical) involves the treatment of individuals with mental or emotional illness.

Forensic psychiatry in America typically does not deal with treatment except in correctional institutions and forensic psychiatric hospitals, but rather with clinical assessment of individuals in criminal or civil cases. The forensic expert may be called either by the prosecution, the defense or the court in a criminal case, or by the plaintiff, the defense or the court in a civil case, or by either side in an administrative legal case. It is usually best for the forensic expert not to be the treating psychiatrist. The goal of treatment is to help the patient, and the goal of forensic psychiatry is to seek justice and truth while respecting the rights of those who are examined [1].

First, Do No Harm

The ethical credo for treating physicians is *primum non nocere*—first, do no harm. Doctors are not supposed to intentionally or negligently harm patients they treat. Their goal is to alleviate suffering and pain while treating the medical condition. However, it is well known that in the course of treating particular illnesses, patients do suffer as a result of the treatment.

For example, in surgical procedures, patients have pain during the procedure even though they are anesthetized and will have pain following the procedure, requiring analgesic medication, which sometimes can be taken to excess and lead to addiction or habituation. Sometimes the surgical procedure inadvertently or unintentionally results in further damage to the patient. For example, abdominal operations sometimes lead to adhesions, which cause further complications in the future. Surgeons always advise their patients that major operations could result in serious complications or even death. Certainly, neurosurgical operations of the brain could lead to problems of mentation or cognition or even movement of limbs. Nevertheless, the option is either to operate with the risks that are usually known (and some that are unknown or unexpected) or to suffer from the pain and complications of the illness. Often, this is a very difficult choice for many patients who have learned to live with the symptoms of their illness and are uncomfortable making a choice about the unknown that may occur following surgical treatment.

Intentional Harm

Medical treatment then can be painful or harmful even though the intention is to relieve pain and alleviate suffering; never should the doctor intentionally inflict harm on his or her patient.

Of course, there are unusual and rare circumstances when physicians have been found to betray the confidences of their patients or to intentionally inflict harm for reasons that are outside the scope of medical practice. One psychiatrist treating a patient for depression gave whopping doses of lithium for bipolar disorder that caused kidney failure. It was later learned, in the criminal trial, that the psychiatrist wanted to kill the patient in order to free the patient's wife, with whom he had fallen in love, to marry him. This type of intentional harm is extremely rare, but when it occurs, it is a breach of trust between the patient and the doctor and should never be tolerated.

Confidentiality

In psychiatry, maintaining confidentiality is extremely important to the welfare of the patient. Talking about patients' illnesses outside the consultation room could lead to damage or harm to the patient by loss of job, loss of reputation, or other complications that may have been unforeseen by the loose lips of the treating psychiatrist.

There are regulations that guide the release of information about patients. Generally speaking, the treating psychiatrist should never reveal any information about his or her patient without proper legal release such as a court order. Even a subpoena may not be sufficient to release information, unless the court orders it following a hearing. Thus, in psychiatry, maintaining confidentiality is a priority that is rarely violated or breached. However, in general medicine, doctors frequently talk about their patients without concern about the information that is revealed. Especially in high profile individuals, physicians may be very proud of the fact that they are the ones treating these important people and want others to know of their value that is enhanced by being selected to treat the "great and the good."

Psychotherapy

In psychiatry, doctors may say things to patients in therapy in order to stimulate a response or to move them off center to look more clearly at their conflicts and gain insight where cognitive blindness had prevented emotional growth. Making comments that may offend in the name of therapy is done judiciously, but doctors are told never to direct their patient to do various things unless they are therapeutic or helpful. Freud, for example, taught his students to listen and to confront or to analyze, but never to direct patients to specific behaviors. However, Peter Kramer, in his book on *Freud: Inventor of the Modern Mind* [2], writes about Freud's direction to a female patient that she should divorce her husband and marry her former analyst, a disciple of Freud's in New York. The woman followed her great analyst's instructions, divorced her husband, left her family, and married her former analyst, who had divorced his wife. Dr. Kramer notes that after three years, the experiment was not a success and the outcome was tragic for both families. Harm came because of the therapeutic direction, even by Freud. I am sure he did not intend to harm his patient or his former student, but his direction to his patient proved extremely harmful to both families.

Though doctors do not intend purposely to harm their patients, sometimes harm does occur either inadvertently, unexpectedly, or unforeseeably. Malpractice cases are based on negligent care by the physician that leads to harm to the patient. The basis is not preventability, but foreseeability. The harm may have been prevented, but was it expected or foreseeable? Harm may come to the patient either from overt behavior that is negligent or from lack of appropriate action. Some malpractice cases develop on the basis of intentional infliction of harm to the patient when the physician's behavior is clearly improper.

Harm in Clinical Psychiatric Practice

In psychiatry, the use of various medications has proliferated with research demonstrating chemical imbalance in a number of different mental illnesses. Therapy, with medication, has been shown to improve various conditions such as depression or mania, or even schizophrenia. Nevertheless, there are side effects of these medications that need to be minimized wherever possible.

Harm may occur to the patient in everyday clinical psychiatric practice, even when the practitioner follows ethical guidelines, either of the American Psychological Association or the American Psychiatric Association. There are conflicts of interest that occur where ethical propositions put the safety of the community over confidentiality of the doctor–patient relationship (e.g., the Tarasoff case) [3]. Individual patients may be harmed in addition when the practitioner engages in research that advances medicine for the benefit of future patients or is mandated to testify in court about private issues of his patient.

Treating psychiatrists should try to avoid testimony whenever possible, but sometimes courts will order the treating psychiatrist or psychologist to testify either in a criminal or civil case, thus potentially harming the patient in the name of preserving the integrity of the law. When breaching confidentiality as mandated in the Tarasoff case, the therapist violates the patient's confidentiality in order to protect an innocent person in the community from the potential violence of his patient. The Codes of Ethics of both the American Psychological Association [4] and the American Psychiatric Association [5] support the court's mandates in these situations, but the practitioner may be able to minimize the harm caused to his patient by adhering to the Guidelines of the Codes of Ethics of the American Academy of Psychiatry and the Law [6].

Grisso [7] assesses the harm that is done in everyday clinical mental health practice. He states, "We often do things in the normal course of clinical work that require actions that may harm an individual. Examples encountered in everyday clinical practice include:

1. mandated breaches of confidentiality in therapeutic relationships.
2. the use of triage in emergency medicine.
3. engaging in clinical research that sacrifices optimal individualized treatment in favor of medical advances for the benefit of future patients.
4. testifying about personality factors in legal cases (e.g., those of felons in criminal cases or of parents in child protection cases) that may result in deprivation of liberties and significant suffering."

Grisso argues that even though harm may come to people because of what psychologists and psychiatrists do in the course of their treating individuals, they are not necessarily practicing unethically. He states, "They all involve two conditions to show that they are not unethical: First they are within the boundaries of a role that is lawfully prescribed to them by society and second, they all allow one to potentially justify the harm that might be done when weighed against the social consequences if one failed to risk the chances of that harm" [8]. Grisso cites the American Psychological Association Code of Ethics in justifying his argument. He states, "Our professional codes of ethics provide ample room for disagreement among reasonable professionals regarding the weight to be placed on an individual's rights and society's interests in regulating our own conduct ... the mere fact that the psychologist places considerable weight on society's interests and acted in a way that would harm the individual in question does not violate the APA's Code of Ethics" [9].

If Grisso is correct, then there are situations in which the mental health professional may put society's interests before the individual's in a way that may cause harm to the individual and still not be improper or unethical. An example is the Tarasoff case in which the therapist has to violate a patient's confidentiality in order to protect those in the community from the potential violence of his patient [3].

Minimizing Harm

Much has been written about the ethics of medicine and, more recently, the ethics of psychiatry and forensic psychiatry [6]. Generally, the ethical prohibition of *primum non nocere*—first, do no harm—applies to medicine generally and to psychiatry specifically. It does not, and cannot, apply to forensic psychiatry, because there is an inherent harm built into the practice of forensic psychiatry within the adversarial system of justice. Even though we may not use *primum non nocere* as the hallmark or guide for forensic psychiatry, we can use the model of minimizing harm in forensic psychiatry.

Psychiatrists know that their assessment of a particular individual, the report they write, or the testimony given will be harmful to certain people. The psychiatrist evaluating a defendant for the prosecution, who determines there is no mental illness and no insanity, knows that a guilty finding will lead to imprisonment in many cases. The psychiatrist may also recognize that, in capital cases, his or her testimony could result in the defendant getting the death penalty.

In civil cases, the psychiatrist examining a plaintiff for the defense, finding no evidence for mental illness or no connection between symptomatology and the alleged incident, knows that the plaintiff will be harmed by not receiving a judgment or an award and may not receive needed treatment as a result.

Bias

Mostly, psychiatrists recognize that they are but a cog in the wheel of justice and their testimony may be important, but not always dispositive. They feel they must be honest and testify to the truth as they see it within their expertise. Many will say they do not concern themselves with the legal outcome, but merely give the opinions they believe are valid and honest for that particular case.

This raises the question of bias, or prejudice, in forensic work. Many years ago, one of the pioneers of modern forensic psychiatry, Dr. Bernard Diamond [10], wrote a masterful article on the fallacy of the impartial expert witness. He had indicated that he would never work for the prosecution, because he thought that was unethical for him. He believed, and so wrote, that all forensic experts have an inherent bias that shows up in their work, and they must be aware of it and discuss it whenever possible.

His contemporary, Dr. Seymour Pollack [11], also recognized the biases that we all have, but claimed that it was something we could recognize, admit to, and still give honest and truthful testimony. He wrote that forensic psychiatry was the profession that met the ends and purposes of the law. He differentiated between the medical examination and the forensic psychiatric examination. Medical examinations are to be conducted in order to come to a diagnosis so the person can receive proper treatment. The forensic examination is part of an overall assessment within the structure of the legal system; conclusions are utilized for the sake of legal purposes rather than medical ones.

Medical v. Legal

Thus, in a medical examination, the diagnosis of schizophrenia is made in order to provide proper treatment and/or medication. In a criminal case, the diagnosis would be utilized in order to justify the conclusion that at the time of the commission of the act in question, the person was suffering from a psychotic illness that prevented him from knowing what he was doing or from knowing that it was wrong. The examination, evaluation, and assessment is not conducted primarily in order to treat the individual, but rather to come to a conclusion that can be utilized in a court of law.

Ethics in Forensic Psychiatry

It is for these reasons that the ethical mandates for forensic psychiatry differ from those in treatment psychiatry. Paul Appelbaum [1] has written that forensic psychiatrists seek justice and must respect the individual being examined. His general concepts have led to the specific behavior by all forensic examiners who act ethically when they alert the person being examined at the beginning of the session, who they are, whom they represent, what they will be doing when they examine the individual, what they will do with the information they receive, how that information might affect the individual, and offer the person to be examined the choice of refusing the examination.

In addition, the person examined must be told that the examination is not for treatment purposes and the examiner will not be treating the person examined. Further, the examinee should be told there can be no traditional doctor–patient confidentiality since a report will be prepared and sent to the retaining attorney or to the judge and will be distributed to the parties involved in the lawsuit or the criminal case.

It is for these reasons that the American Academy of Psychiatry and the Law has developed guidelines for ethical work in forensic psychiatry [6]. These ethical guidelines support the notion of confidentiality and limited confidentiality and emphasize that the ethical forensic psychiatrist will strive for neutrality and objectivity. They utilize the words *strive for* because they recognize that there cannot be an absolute objectivity or neutrality. The forensic psychiatrist can certainly achieve honesty to the best of his or her ability. Achieving neutrality and objectivity, however, is more difficult, because of the inherent bias and the pressures on the individual expert within the adversarial system.

One test of neutrality and objectivity is the track record of the expert in terms of his or her working for the prosecution and finding the defendant either to be incompetent or to meet the test of legal insanity in that jurisdiction. In how many cases has that occurred in the expert's history? Similarly, how many times has the defense expert found no evidence for incompetency or insanity in the cases he or she has assessed and evaluated?

Another test of objectivity and neutrality is the manner in which the expert may assess, either for the prosecution or defense in criminal cases, or for the defendant or the plaintiff in civil cases. Another test will be how many times a judge, who serves as the gatekeeper for testimony, will call upon the expert, because the expert has a reputation for seeking truth and justice and appears neutral and objective, utilizing scientific evidence to support his or her opinions and conclusions rather than speculation or bias.

Another test of objectivity is the number of times that both attorneys, one on either side, will agree to a particular expert examining the plaintiff in civil cases, or the defendant in criminal cases, and agree to abide by the opinion reached by the expert psychiatrist.

Dual Agency

Alan Stone [12] is concerned about dual agency, and cautions that the psychiatrist, even when he gives what I have referred to as "Psychiatric Miranda Warnings," explaining to the examinee who he is, whom he represents, and what he will do with the information he obtains, can still be seen by the examinee as a physician who is there to do good rather than to seek the truth. He is concerned that there is a built-in seductive quality to the examiner which means that the examinee will forget about the warnings after a few hours of questioning.

I agree with Dr. Stone that one can be extremely seductive to a suspicious defendant who has usually been lied to by others, or betrayed, or questioned with hostility and in an accusatory tone. The psychiatrist, who comes across as sincere and reveals his respect for the examinee, can get much more information from the individual than one who is challenging, hostile, and cynical. Is it fair to the examinee to be confronted by such a skillful, talented, and sincere psychiatrist who is seeking the truth and may allow the normal guardedness of the examinee to be minimized so that further information is obtained by such examination?

Certainly, there are individuals who are so guarded, they will tell the examiner very little or nothing, especially at the beginning. Why should a defendant tell a psychiatrist hired by the prosecution his innermost secrets when he is told that the psychiatrist is going to put that in a report and send it to the defendant's enemy, that is, the prosecutor, who is seen by the defendant as one who wants to find him guilty so that he can punish and/or imprison him?

Attorneys Help Minimize Harm

Safeguards have been developed within the system to prevent exploitation of the defendant by skilled psychiatric examiners. For example, it is prohibited for a forensic psychiatrist to examine a person charged with crime before that person has an attorney retained or appointed for him. Clearly, if the defendant is seriously mentally ill and requires treatment on an emergency basis, a psychiatrist may come in to conduct an examination in order to make a diagnosis so that proper treatment can be rendered to ease the mental and emotional pain and suffering. However, what is learned in the course of that assessment may not be used against the defendant in his criminal case.

Similarly, once an attorney has been retained or appointed, that attorney may advise his client not to talk to anyone about the case. The attorney will advise his client to speak directly to his expert, and will often do so after being properly introduced by the attorney. However, the attorney may tell his client not to talk to the psychiatrist appointed by the prosecution. That had been more frequent in prior cases, but more recently, courts have disallowed defense attorneys to proceed with an insanity defense unless they allow the prosecution to have their expert examine the defendant. Sometimes, the defense will ask the court to order the prosecution expert's examination to be videotaped or will want the expert defense psychiatrist present during the examination by the prosecution expert. The prosecution expert may object, saying that he was not allowed or invited to be present when the defense psychiatrist examined the defendant, so he does not want the defense expert to be present during his examination. He may have no choice if the judge orders the defense psychiatrist to be present.

Minimizing Harm

This book is not about medicine or treating psychiatry, but rather about the inherent harm that may be caused in the practice of forensic psychiatry. Forensic psychiatrists do not have the mandate of "First, Do No Harm." Their mandate is to seek truth and justice and to aid the legal process by striving for neutrality and objectivity, irrespective of which side of the adversary system they represent. As Appelbaum has so aptly stated, one of our ethical goals is to show respect for the individual [1]. This means not only telling the examinee who we are, whom we represent, what we will do with the information we glean from the individual, but maintaining the confidentiality to a limited degree. By that, I mean we should not reveal information to anyone but the retaining attorney, who may then choose to distribute our reports or the information given to appropriate individuals. There are exceptions, of course, when there is a court order or a valid subpoena for the records. It is usually better not to send the records to the examinee. I have occasionally been asked by the examinee's therapist or subsequent examiner to forward my information to the treating psychiatrist or psychologist. With a letter from that therapist and a signed release of information from the examinee, I will release the information. If treating doctors wish to share that information with the persons examined, that is their prerogative and the responsibility of any untoward reaction is on them.

These are all important issues in our consideration of conducting assessments and evaluations that may cause harm. There are many different ways of practicing forensic psychiatry based on one's personal bias, personal experiences and observations of the examinee's behavior. These differences may account for the different opinions or opposite opinions that various forensic psychiatrists may give regarding the same individual under the same circumstances. In evaluating why experts may cause harm during their forensic assessments, including the examination, report writing, and testimony, we have to look at the experiences of the expert, the moral and ethical values held by the mental health professional, and the observations made during the course of the examination. All of these differences may account for the variability often seen in forensic psychiatry that has stimulated skepticism on the part of non-forensic psychiatrists about the reliability, validity, and credibility of forensic psychiatric practice.

Finally, it is, therefore, respect for the individual that is necessary in minimizing harm to those who are involved in the adversarial system of justice. We may not be able to totally eliminate harm, but we can certainly be sensitive to the potential for damage to our evaluees and make every effort to minimize or limit the harm that can occur to those individuals caught in the legal system of justice.

References

1. Appelbaum, P.S. (1997) A theory of ethics for forensic psychiatry. *Journal of the American Academy of Psychiatry and the Law*, **25**, 233–47.
2. Kramer, P.D. (2006) *Freud: Inventor of the Modern Mind*. Atlas Books, Harper Collins, New York.
3. *Tarasoff v. Board of Regents of University of California*, 551 P.2d 334(Cal.) (1976).
4. Committee on Ethical Guidelines for Forensic Psychologists (1991) Specialty guidelines for forensic psychologists. *Law and Human Behavior*, **15**, 6.
5. The American Psychiatric Association (2008) *The Principles of Medical Ethics, with Annotations especially Applicable to Psychiatry*. Washington, DC.
6. The American Academy of Psychiatry and the Law (2005) *Ethics Guidelines for the Practice of Forensic Psychiatry*. Bloomfield, CT.
7. Grisso, T. (2001) Reply to Schafer: doing harm ethically. *Journal of the American Academy of Psychiatry and the Law*, **29**, 457–60.
8. See Ref. [7] at p. 458.
9. See Ref. [7] at p. 460.
10. Diamond, B. (1959) The fallacy of the impartial expert. *Archives of Criminal Psychodynamics*, **3**, 221.
11. Pollack, S.D. (1974) *Psychiatry in Criminal Law*. University of Southern California Press, Los Angeles.
12. Stone, A.A. (1984) The ethical boundaries of forensic psychiatry: a view from the ivory tower. *Bulletin of the American Academy of Psychiatry and the Law*, **12**, 209–19.

List of Contributors

John A. Baird, MD, FRCPsych DCH
Consultant Forensic Psychiatrist
Leverndale Hospital,
Glasgow, Scotland, UK

Solange Margery Bertoglia, MD
Assistant Professor of Psychiatry
Thomas Jefferson University Hospital,
Philadelphia, PA, USA

Luis Fernando Barrios Flores, JD
Department of State Legal Studies
University of Alicante,
Alicante, Spain

Emanuele Valenti, PhD
Associate Professor of Medical Humanities and Bioethics
Medical School,
European University of Madrid,
Madrid, Spain

Donna L. Vanderpool, MBA, JD
Assistant Vice President, Risk Management
Professional Risk Management Services, Inc.
Arlington, VA, USA

Part One

Ethics in Forensic Psychiatry

1 Ethical Issues in Forensic Psychiatry in the United States

Robert L. Sadoff

University of Pennsylvania School of Medicine, Philadelphia, USA

1.1 Introduction

The forensic psychiatrist or psychologist works within the judicial system, which is not a therapeutic system. Rather, the judicial system is one that seeks truth and justice, irrespective of harm that may come either to the defendant in a criminal case, or the plaintiff in a civil case or an individual in an administrative legal case.

The criminal justice system seeks to punish those who are guilty of criminal behavior. In civil matters, the court attempts to seek justice by awarding damages to those who have been harmed by others. The court also attempts to identify those who are not harmed, but claim to be. Forensic mental health experts are utilized by the judicial system to aid in the process of discovery and adjudication. Thus, the forensic psychiatrist may find him or herself working within a system that is not therapeutic and may cause significant harm to various individuals. How can the forensic medical expert work within such a system while adhering to the ethical tenets of our profession and not causing harm to those with whom we work?

We have already established that the major ethical issue in medicine is "first, do no harm." We have also shown that patients are indeed harmed in the name of therapy, even in the course of conducting diagnostic procedures. With the intention of helping patients, we may often harm them. In psychiatry, we have also shown that patients can be harmed either with medication, somatic treatment modalities or even psychotherapy.

In the Preamble to the *Principles of Medical Ethics* of the American Medical Association (AMA), the AMA affirms that "The medical profession has long

Ethical Issues in Forensic Psychiatry: Minimizing Harm   by Robert L. Sadoff
© 2011 John Wiley & Sons, Ltd

subscribed to a body of ethical statements developed primarily for the benefit of the patient. As a member of this profession, a physician must recognize responsibility to patients first and foremost, as well as to society, to other health professionals, and to self"[1]. The following list outlines the major principles that have been adopted by the American Medical Association. They are not considered laws, but are "standards of conduct which define the essentials of honorable behavior for the physician."[1]

1. A physician shall be dedicated to providing competent medical service with compassion and respect for human dignity.
2. A physician shall deal honestly with patients and colleagues, and strive to expose those physicians deficient in character or competence or who engage in fraud or deception.
3. A physician shall respect the law and also recognize a responsibility to seek changes in those requirements which are contrary to the best interests of the patient.
4. A physician shall respect the rights of patients, of colleagues, and of other health professionals, and shall safeguard patients' confidences within the constraints of the law.
5. A physician shall continue to study, apply, and advance scientific knowledge, make relevant information available to patients, colleagues, and the public, obtain consultation, and use the talents of other health professionals when indicated.
6. A physician shall in the provision of appropriate patient care, except in emergencies, be free to choose whom to serve, with whom to associate, and the environment in which to provide medical services.
7. A physician shall recognize the responsibility to participate in activities contributing to an improved community.

Clearly, the concept of *primum non nocere* cannot apply to forensic psychiatric practice. There are inherent harms that can be caused either during the examination, the report writing or the testimony given in forensic cases. The forensic examiner must alert the examinee that he will not be treating him, and there can be no traditional doctor-patient confidentiality. In essence, there is no doctor-patient relationship developed, because there is no agreement for treatment. The examiner is appointed either by the examinee's attorney, by an attorney for the other side, or by the judge to conduct the examination. Irrespective of who retains the examiner, he or she may inflict damage on the examinee. Thus, there is no prohibition in forensic cases to not do harm as there is in treatment cases in medicine generally, and in psychiatry in particular.

In many cases, there is harm done in forensic mental health matters. This is usually not intentional harm, but it is harm that is built in to the adversarial system in which the forensic psychiatrist works. We have discussed the bias that may exist that could lead to harmful examinations, harmful statements in the report, or harmful comments during testimony. The purpose of this presentation is to alert forensic experts about such potential harm and to attempt to minimize, limit, or eliminate, if possible, the harm that can be caused by the forensic expert.

1.2 AAPL Guidelines

Forensic psychiatrists have recognized that they cannot utilize the time-tested ethical prohibition against doing harm as their mantra in ethical practice, but must formulate ethical conditions that are more appropriate to the forensic setting. As a result, the American Academy of Psychiatry and the Law (AAPL) developed a set of guidelines that were initiated in the mid-1970s. The first attempt occurred when three members of the Academy sat down to attempt to formulate guidelines for forensic practitioners.[1] Those guidelines underwent several modifications that were published as official actions of AAPL until the most recent, in 2005, which have been published by the AAPL [2].

In these guidelines, forensic psychiatry is defined as follows: It is "a subspecialty of psychiatry in which scientific and clinical expertise is applied in legal contexts involving civil, criminal, correctional, regulatory, or legislative matters, and in specialized clinical consultations in areas such as risk assessment or employment. These guidelines apply to psychiatrists practicing in a forensic role" [2]. I have defined forensic psychiatry as the subspecialty of psychiatry that deals with people who are involved in legal matters, either criminal or civil. Clearly, the definition in the AAPL guidelines is much more comprehensive, but less understood by juries when the expert is asked to define forensic psychiatry in court.

The AAPL has clearly indicated that their guidelines "supplement the *Annotations Especially Applicable to Psychiatry* of the American Psychiatric Association to the principles of medical ethics of the American Medical Association" [2]. The APA guidelines state clearly that "psychiatrists in a forensic role are called upon to practice in a manner that balances competing duties to the individual and to society. In doing so, they should be bound by ethical principles of respect for persons, honesty, justice, and social responsibility. However, when a treatment relationship exists, such as in correctional settings, the usual physician-patient duties apply" [3]. Generally, the AAPL guidelines comment on issues of confidentiality, consent, honesty, and striving for objectivity, and the qualifications of the expert.

1.3 Appelbaum's Concepts

It should be noted that many of these concepts within the guidelines stem from the brilliant paper of Paul Appelbaum that appeared in the *Journal of AAPL*

---

[1] In the mid-1970s, Drs. Jonas Rappeport, Irwin Perr, and Robert Sadoff wrote the first draft of what is now the *Ethics Guidelines for the Practice of Forensic Psychiatry* by the American Academy of Psychiatry and the Law, adopted in May 2005.

in 1997, entitled, "A theory of ethics for forensic psychiatry". In the introduction, Appelbaum states,

> This article offers a justification for a set of principles that constitute the ethical underpinnings of forensic psychiatry. For forensic psychiatrists, the primary value of their work is to advance the interests of justice. The two principles on which that effort rests are truth telling and respect for persons [4].

A virtue of this approach is the clear distinction it offers between forensic and therapeutic roles.

Thus, Appelbaum alludes to the issue of working for justice and truth and respect for the individual who is examined. In that context of respect, the forensic expert must tell the examinee who he or she is, whom he represents, what will happen during the examination, what are the consequences to the examinee of such an examination (for example, can the defendant in a capital case, get the death penalty if the defendant cooperates with the forensic psychiatrist appointed by the prosecution?). Nevertheless, the evaluator must give this information to the examinee in order for the person examined to give informed consent for the examination. Anything less would not be respect for the individual examined.

The idea of searching for truth implies a degree of neutrality and objectivity in the examination. The ethics guidelines by AAPL indicate that we should be "striving for" neutrality and objectivity, inasmuch as it may never be totally reached because of the human element of bias, errors, and other factors that cloud the issue and inhibit the totality of objectivity.

Others have argued that the guidelines should be more compelling and eliminate the words "striving for" and push for total objectivity and neutrality.[2] It would be nice to have such an ideal situation, but if it cannot be implemented, then it is an ideal that is not practical. We should set the goals for guidelines in ethics in forensic psychiatry to those which can be practiced and implemented.

Thus, in my opinion, Appelbaum has laid the groundwork for the guidelines that have evolved through several modifications of the AAPL Committee on Ethics [2]. The 2005 guidelines are workable, practical, and should be recognized as the accepted ethics for forensic psychiatrists conducting their examinations, preparing their reports, and offering testimony that affect individuals involved in the judicial system.

1.4 Confidentiality

The guidelines refer to confidentiality, which is an ethical proposition within medicine generally. I have often found the guideline for confidentiality in general medicine to be honored more in the breach than in its acceptance. Psychiatrists tend to be more protective of the privacy of their communications with their patients than physicians in general. In forensic work, there is a limitation to confidentiality that must be discussed with the examinee at the outset of the examination. The

---

[2] Personal communications from several members of AAPL.

examinee must be told that there will be a report prepared and sent to the retaining attorney, whether it be the defendant's own attorney, or the prosecutor in criminal cases, or the plaintiff's attorney, or the defense attorney in civil cases.

There are a number of attempts to invade the privacy or confidentiality of these medical records. For example, the examinee has often asked that a copy of the records be sent to him or her. I have never sent records directly to the individual examined for a number of reasons. First, the patient may not be able to accept the concepts without being harmed, unless they are read to him and explained to him by his therapist. By definition, I, the forensic examiner, am not his therapist and cannot accept the role of explaining my observations, impressions, or opinions to him in a therapeutic context, because that would blur my role. I have sent the records, when requested with a signed release of information to the individual's therapist, who can then discuss the report with the individual in a therapeutic context.

Generally, I send the report only to the retaining attorney and know that the attorney will be distributing the report to others, and may even send it directly to the attorney's client. If that is the case, the attorney then assumes responsibility for the consequences of his distributing the report. A number of attorneys will refuse to give the report to their clients, believing the client is too fragile or may "freak out" when reading the report. A number of examinees have called to try to get the report directly from me when they cannot get it from their attorney. It is always good conduct and a wise decision to call the attorney to determine why he or she does not send the report directly to the person examined. One of the reasons is the fragility of the examinee, but another may be that the client has not paid the attorney's bill, and the attorney is withholding the report until he is paid. We would not want to interfere in any way with the attorney-client relationship by providing the report in such cases where the client has not been faithful to his own attorney.

At some later date, on a post-conviction appeal (PCRA) an attorney may request the records in order to show that his client did not have effective assistance of counsel and his conviction should be overturned. In those cases, a subpoena will be issued to the forensic expert to receive his report and any supporting data that was utilized in reaching his opinions. How long should the psychiatrist retain his records? My practice is to strip my file after the conclusion of the case in chief. I keep the records that I generated for 7–10 years, and then discard them, because the law allows us to do so. However, for the first 10 years, I will keep my report and correspondence in the file that may be necessary for some future use. Sometimes, I receive requests for records that are 20 or 30 years old, and I just don't have them. I often assume that attorneys will keep the supporting data they have sent to me for my review. However, the original attorney may not wish to cooperate with the appellate attorney who is criticizing his work. That becomes an issue between the attorneys and the forensic psychiatrist should not be placed in an awkward position to intrude on that relationship.

In summary, it is wise to restrict the distribution of the report from the forensic psychiatrist only to the retaining attorney, who will then distribute it according to his or her legal requirements. It is also essential that the examinee be alerted to the limitation on confidentiality since most individuals believe that what they tell a psychiatrist is secret or private, and that cannot be the case in forensic work.

1.5 Informed Consent

The next ethical issue is that of consent, and that involves alerting the evaluee about what will be done with the information gleaned and what effect it will have upon the person examined. In addition, I may need to testify at a hearing or in court about what I learned in the course of the examination. The examinee should be told that such disclosure may need to occur and that I could not keep secret what he told me. He needs to be forewarned about what would happen to the information so that he can give proper informed consent to the examination.

It is also important that the information given to the person examined before he or she divulges any information should include what possible consequences could occur to him or her in that particular case. An example is the case of *Barefoot v. Estelle* [5], a Texas case in which the Supreme Court overturned the guilty verdict because the expert who gave the information to the defendant did not divulge that his testimony could result in the defendant receiving the death penalty.

People have a right not to cooperate with the forensic psychiatrist, and many will not do so for a number of reasons. I have had individuals balk at speaking with me because they were told by their attorney that I was a neurologist and not a psychiatrist. They asked the question, "What does my attorney think, I'm nuts?" They refuse to cooperate until they have a chance to talk with their attorney and clarify the reason for the examination and my role. Sometimes, when visiting an individual in prison, the defendant will not speak with me unless his attorney is present, and that needs to be arranged at some later date. I always give the defendant the benefit of the doubt and allow him to refuse to cooperate until his attorney is alerted and they can work out a solution that is least harmful to the defendant.

1.6 Competency

The issue of competency to consent is raised in the AAPL guidelines. Sometimes, the defendant, in a criminal case, or the plaintiff, in a civil case, is not competent to give consent to the examination. In those cases, there should be others at the examination to give consent for the individual examined. For example, in a civil case, the individual examined may be so injured that the brain damage limits his ability to cooperate or to even give consent to the examination. The examination may be conducted in order to determine his competency in this matter, and the extent of damage that can be assessed if permission is given by a legally appointed surrogate or a guardian.

In criminal cases, the issue of competency is often assessed at various stages of the criminal proceedings. A person who is not competent to stand trial may be competent to give consent to the examination in order to determine his competency to proceed. In the event that he is not competent to give consent, his attorney should be present to protect his rights.

A clear example of this occurred about 30 years ago, in Philadelphia, when three mental health professionals were appointed by the court to evaluate a criminal defendant for the prosecution. There were two psychiatrists and a psychologist, all of whom had experience in working in the criminal justice system. In those days, the defendant did not have to cooperate with experts for the prosecution even if he planned to present an insanity defense. In this particular case, the defendant, standing 6′ 7″ and weighing over 300 pounds, was very specific in his statement to the three of us, that he refused to cooperate with the court-appointed experts for the prosecution and respectfully would not give any statement to us. The two psychiatrists were prepared to leave when the psychologist inappropriately (and, in my opinion, unethically and foolishly) challenged the defendant, who was sitting with his attorney and with us in a private room. The psychologist said that if the defendant did not speak with us, the psychologist might consider him to be incompetent and he would, therefore, be detained in the mental health system indefinitely until he could cooperate and could be deemed competent to proceed.

At that point, I intervened, telling the psychologist, with great passion, that he must retract his statement, apologize to the defendant, and that we would leave peacefully and not make any further threats. I was not only concerned about the unethical manner in which he threatened the defendant, but I was also concerned about our physical safety. The psychologist was easily convinced that it was in everyone's best interest for him to apologize and for us to withdraw before there was violence. I also added to the defendant that we were sorry about the psychologist's comments and that we would not, and could not, make any statement about his competency. We would merely report to the judge that the defendant "respectfully refused to cooperate with us." It would then be up to the judge to determine the next step in the proceedings.

The AAPL guidelines commentary on informed consent discusses various exceptions and special cases. They note that, in particular situations, "such as court-ordered evaluations for competency to stand trial or involuntary commitment, neither assent nor informed consent is required. In such cases, psychiatrists should inform the evaluee that if the evaluee refuses to participate in the evaluation, this fact may be included in any report or testimony. If the evaluee does not appear capable of understanding the information provided regarding the evaluation, this impression should also be included in any report and, when feasible, in testimony" [2].

1.7   Presence of Legal Counsel

Further to the commentary, the guidelines note that "absent a court order, psychiatrists should not perform forensic evaluations for the prosecution or the government on persons who have not consulted with legal counsel when such persons are known to be charged with criminal acts; under investigation for criminal or quasi-criminal conduct; held in government custody or detention; or being interrogated for criminal or quasi-criminal conduct, hostile acts against government, or immigration violations. Examinations related to rendering medical care or treatment, such as evaluations for civil commitment or risk assessments for management or discharge planning, are not precluded by these restrictions. As is true for any physician, psychiatrists practicing in a forensic role should not participate in torture" [2].

The long statement precluding assessment of individuals in quasi-criminal situations from being evaluated without the advice of legal counsel stems from examples of individuals who were examined by forensic psychiatrists upon arrest and before counsel could be obtained. Without the advice of counsel, a number of these individuals gave statements they would not have given had they been properly advised by their attorneys. The prohibition to forensic psychiatrists is that we do not cooperate with the state inappropriately by tricking or deceiving the individual before he has proper advice from his attorney so that he can be protected under the law and the Constitution. Psychiatrists should not be agents of the state in promoting deception or torture in order to get information from the defendant. This would be clearly unethical. However, individuals newly arrested, who have serious mental problems, may be in need of emergency treatment, which is appropriate and may be given. Those treating psychiatrists should then be precluded from ever testifying against the defendant at a later date.

1.8 Objectivity, Honesty, and Neutrality

Under the concept of striving for objectivity and neutrality, the commentary indicates "The adversarial nature of most legal processes presents special hazards for the practice of forensic psychiatry. Being retained by one side in a civil or criminal matter exposes psychiatrists to the potential for unintended bias and the danger of distortion of their opinion. It is the responsibility of psychiatrists to minimize such hazards by acting in an honest manner and striving to reach an objective opinion." [6].

The early attempts by the AAPL Committee on Ethics to develop guidelines also included concepts of neutrality, honesty, and striving for objectivity when conducting forensic psychiatric examinations. The committee recognized that one could not always achieve total neutrality or objectivity, but at least the attempt was made to strive for such an ideal. The committee was clearly influenced by Bernard Diamond's seminal paper on the "Fallacy of the impartial expert" [7], recognizing that all assessors have inherent biases that need to be recognized. Seymour Pollack [8], one of the early pioneers in modern forensic psychiatry, had cautioned that recognizing our biases is important, and they must be "put on the table" when we are involved in forensic cases.

1.9 Cultural Differences

Ezra E.H. Griffith, in his article, "Ethics in forensic psychiatry: A cultural response to Stone and Appelbaum" [9], focuses on the cultural differences and critiques

Stone and Appelbaum positing the notion that it is important for the assessor to have a cultural knowledge of the person being interviewed and evaluated. He has stated that it would be more equitable for the African American criminal defendant to be examined by an African American forensic psychiatrist, who would understand the nuances of his cultural situation, rather than by a Caucasian forensic psychiatrist, who may not have understanding of the cultural background.

Griffith continues by stating, "I'm concerned about the unwitting collusion to exclude the voices of the non-dominant groups . . . A theoretical ethics framework is not persuasive if it merely brings orderliness into the sustained interaction of dominant and non-dominant group members, while preserving the traditional higher ethical relationship between the groups" [10].

Ciccone and Clements [11] support the notion that there are cultural differences that must be accounted for in the ethical principles governing forensic psychiatry and forensic examinations.

Hicks, in his paper, "Ethnicity, race, and forensic psychiatry: are we color blind?" [12] advises that forensic psychiatrists and psychologists should consider race, ethnicity, and culture when performing evaluations for legal purposes and when providing treatment to the special populations with whom they work. Hicks notes, "Findings in several studies have shown that African Americans are more often diagnosed with psychosis and whites with mood disorders in emergency rooms and at hospitalization . . . elderly African Americans are more frequently given diagnoses of psychotic disorders and dementia . . . than are elderly whites."

Hicks is also concerned about the assessment for dangerousness and states that psychiatrists show a higher level of "dangerousness" with minorities than with whites. He declares, "There is an imprecision and ample room for clinicians' bias to influence the decisions with serious consequences. According to the 1990 General Social Survey of Public Perceptions, respondents were more likely to identify African Americans and Hispanics as prone to violence" [13].

As an example of the disparity from a racial standpoint, Lykken states, "From 1973 to 1980, cases involving an African American defendant and white victim were more than seven times more likely to result in the death penalty than cases involving a white defendant and an African American victim" [14]. He also notes that there is an unfairness in the diversion of offenders to substance abuse and mental health treatment between and among whites and African Americans. He concludes that studies have shown that white adolescents with behavioral problems "tend to end up in the mental health system, whereas African American adolescents exhibiting similar behavior end up in the criminal justice system." Lykken is also concerned about the expert witness in examining a person of different ethnic or racial background and states, "The forensic evaluator may experience fear, unease, or identification with the subject. The subject may be more suspicious and mistrustful of a white evaluator, who might be perceived as an instrument of the majority-dominated justice or mental health systems. The subject may also have unrealistic expectations of favorable treatment from an evaluator who belongs to an ethnic and minority group" [14].

Similarly, Griffith states, "Expert witnesses must be vigilant in monitoring their own potential biases. The ethnicity of the forensic psychiatrist, the ethnicity of the subject and the interaction between dominant and non-dominant ethnic groups in the justice system may all affect an examiner's neutrality in complicated ways" [9]. In summary, Griffith is concerned that the non-dominant minority defendant in a criminal case may be harmed if he is examined by an insensitive, dominant forensic psychiatrist who is not aware of the cultural nuances that may significantly affect the examination and the legal conclusions.

In his discussion of the bias that may be inherent in our work, and especially when there is a cultural difference, Silva states, "We need to be able to view the total environment, perhaps as seen by those whom we examine rather than by those who have taught us the abstract system of justice and truth. We need to understand the issues that face the defendant or the plaintiff and how they view our role and our conclusions" [15].

Reid, in his paper, "Ethics and forensic work" [16], discusses various ethical issues for the forensic psychiatrist and is primarily concerned about bias. He states we should do our best to recognize and set aside our significant biases. His major concern is knowingly allowing bias to control testimony. Reid declares, "Bias for a particular view or opinion is just as problematic as bias against it, and arguably more subtle. The witness stand is not the place to express your philosophy nor to allow your philosophy to shape, substantially at least, your opinions in a case ... Testimony is rarely an appropriate vehicle for pressing one's personal or philosophical views" [16].

Reid is also concerned about the psychiatrist working outside of his area of expertise. He writes about a young psychiatrist who had accepted a forensic referral and "told the attorney calling him that he understood the general rules of forensic work." During deposition on cross examination, "he was asked if he had taken notes during the many hours of interviewing various people. The expert said he had, but that he had shredded his notes upon receiving the deposition subpoena." Reid notes that this "was not only imprudent, but arguably an illegal act that belied the witnesses' earlier representation to the authority that he was competent to be an expert. His testimony ruined his usefulness in the case and wasted the attorney's and the plaintiff's time and money" [17].

1.10 Competency

These issues raise the question of the expertise of the forensic examiner. There are a number of general psychiatrists who become involved in legal matters without proper training or experience. Some do not know the specific criteria required for determining a person's competency since the determination will vary depending on the reason the person is examined. For example, one may be competent for one particular event, but not for another.

An example that I often use is the elderly female who is examined in a nursing home for competency to prepare a will. The woman may be competent to prepare her will or sign the will inasmuch as she understands generally how much money she has and to whom she can leave the money if she chooses. However, she may not know what things cost, she may be of weakened intellect and be victimized by designing persons who may steal from her because she is not competent to handle her own affairs. Thus, one should always pose the question about competency: competent for what purpose?

With respect to competency, there are varying rules that govern one's examination and expert opinion. They vary in different jurisdictions and, of course, they vary depending on the purpose of the examination. As an example, New Jersey has specific criteria for competency to stand trial,

"No person that lacks capacity to understand the proceedings against him or to assist in his own defense shall be tried, convicted, or sentenced for the commission of an offense so long as such incapacity endures."

A person shall be considered mentally competent to stand trial on criminal charges if the proofs shall establish:

- that the defendant has the mental capacity to appreciate his presence in relation to time, place, and things;
- that his elementary mental processes are such that he comprehends:
- that he is in a court of justice charged with a criminal offense;
- that there is a judge on the bench;
- that there is a prosecutor present who will try to convict him of a criminal charge;
- that he has a lawyer who will undertake to defend him against that charge;
- that he will be expected to tell to the best of his mental ability the facts surrounding him at the time and place where the alleged violation was committed if he chooses to testify and understands the right not to testify;
- that there is or may be a jury present to pass upon evidence adduced as to guilt or innocence of such charge or, that if he should choose to enter into plea negotiations or to plead guilty, that he comprehend the consequences of a guilty plea and that he be able to knowingly, intelligently, and voluntarily waive those rights which are waived upon such entry of a guilty plea; and
- "that he has the ability to participate in an adequate presentation of his defense."[3]

1.11   Clinical Case Examples

In keeping with the cultural differences that may result in harm if one does not understand cultural nuances, I can offer two examples from my own practice.

In one case, I was asked to examine a criminal defendant in another country who had a different culture and a different language from my own. He had been charged with murder. I had no knowledge of his culture and told the defense attorney that before becoming involved in the case, I would need to study the culture of that country. Indeed, when there, I not only examined the defendant for several hours over many days, but I also interviewed the elders of his culture

---

[3] New Jersey Statutes 2A:163-2, Model Penal Code: 4.04 Amended 1 1979, c. 178, sec. 13.

and had a mock jury of them to determine their cultural view of the defendant's behavior. That was extremely helpful in reaching my opinion that I rendered in a report to the defense attorney.

In another case, in examining, for the prosecution, a woman who had been charged with the death of her newborn baby (neonaticide), I determined that the woman had just come from Mexico, did not speak English, and had been in the United States less than a week when the baby was born and had died. In the course of conducting the examination after about one hour, the Spanish-English translator said to me, "I don't know who I'm speaking with." By that, she meant the defendant had switched, as in dissociative identity disorder (DID), and had become an alter who spoke in a different tone, using a different approach that was not consistent with what had occurred during the first hour of the examination. I immediately stopped the examination and called the prosecutor, telling him that I could not continue in the best interest of justice, because one would need to have a Spanish-speaking forensic psychiatrist in order to determine the nuances of the mental disorder that appeared to be occurring at that time. I never did learn whether she had a DID or what the legal outcome of the case was, but I felt that it was necessary in order to avoid further harm to the defendant (and to justice), that I recuse myself from the case.

With respect to bias, another case occurred in which I was asked by a criminal defense attorney to examine his client, who was a purported Skinhead who had killed his family. I suggested to the attorney that it would not be appropriate for me to conduct the examination, because I could not do it without some prejudice or bias that might affect my objectivity or neutrality. He asked why, and I told him that I was certain that his client would not wish to be examined by a Jewish forensic psychiatrist and that I would have feelings about his view of life and his animosity toward me and my people as well. I suggested we try to find an ethnically neutral forensic psychiatrist (which we were able to do, but only with great difficulty).

1.12   Evidence-Based Psychiatry

Further, the guidelines indicate that the work of forensic psychiatrists should be based upon evidence that can support their opinions. The guidelines state, "They communicate the honesty of their work, efforts to obtain objectivity, and the soundness of their clinical opinion, by distinguishing, to the extent possible, between verified and unverified information as well as among clinical 'facts,' 'inferences,' and 'impressions'" [2].

Several cases have emerged, including Daubert [18] and Kumho [19], replacing Frye [20] in some jurisdictions as standards for presenting testimony in court. Generally, these cases require the judge to be the gatekeeper to limit testimony to that which is based on scientific evidence and not "junk science." The testimony also must be helpful to the trier of fact, whether it be judge or jury.

1.13   Personal Examination

The commentary of AAPL guidelines also indicates a very basic statement, "Psychiatrists should not distort their opinion in the service of the retaining party" [2]. Honesty, objectivity, and the adequacy of the clinical evaluation may be called into question when an expert opinion is offered without a personal examination. The guidelines indicate that an opinion may be rendered on the basis of other information if a personal examination is not available. But the guidelines state, "Under these circumstances, it is the responsibility of psychiatrists to make earnest efforts to insure that their statements, opinions, and any reports or testimony based on these opinions, clearly state that there was no personal examination and note any resulting limitations to their opinions" [2].

Case examples in which a person may not be examined include complex domestic relations cases in which certain individuals or children may not be examined. Sometimes, the examiner in a child custody case is retained by either the mother or father, and the opposite parent refuses to cooperate with that examiner unless he or she is court-ordered. The commentary of AAPL guidelines specifies custody cases which may be very difficult, and in which the psychiatrist must disclose the basis for his opinion and the limitations of the opinion when a full examination could not be conducted [2].

Another example is that of a will contest in which the decedent is evaluated for mental state at a previous time, but, of course, is not available for a direct examination. In those cases, the guidelines indicate that a clear statement must be made about the limitations of the assessment, because no direct examination was made.

1.13.1   Case Example

A man was killed in an automobile accident, and the question was raised whether or not he experienced pain and suffering before he died. The police reports were inadequate to determine whether he suffered prior to his death. In order to attempt to answer the question, I spoke to family members about the kind of person he was and how he viewed his life. I also reviewed the accident scene reports and forensic pathology reports that indicated the victim was conscious prior to his death. Because of his consciousness prior to death and the type of individual he was, it was my opinion, within reasonable medical certainty, that he did experience pain and suffering prior to his death. However, I had to declare in my report and in my testimony that my opinions were limited because I did not examine the individual about whom I was giving an opinion. My opinions were based primarily on reports of others and written reports of professionals.

In another similar matter, there was an airplane crash in which several people were killed, others were badly injured, and many others "walked away without a scratch." In attempting to assess pain and suffering prior to death, it was necessary to review the forensic pathology reports indicating the passengers were conscious for two minutes prior to their death. Utilizing the scientific evidence of the forensic pathologist, I was then able to interview a number of the survivors and their anxiety and other feelings that they experienced prior to the crash, at the time of the crash, and following the crash. I was able to divide the time around the crash into 10 different periods during which the survivors experienced various emotions. Utilizing those data and the forensic pathology reports, I was able to give an opinion, within reasonable medical certainty, that the 10 people who died experienced various emotions, including pain and suffering, for the two minutes they were conscious prior to their losing consciousness and their death. In both cases, it was important to verify in the report that the opinions were based on various information that I had without a direct examination of the victims.

1.13.2 Competency in a Wills Case

In a wills case, in which the records were evaluated after the death of the testator, I noted the examining psychologist reached the opinion that the testator had been depressed and, as a result of depression, was subject to undue influence by others due to a weakened intellect. However, there was a scrivener of the will who testified at deposition that the testator was competent at the time of the writing of the will. The attorney, who was the scrivener, testified that she had tried to influence the decedent into changing her will, but the testator was insistent on having the will written her way. She resisted all efforts to change her mind and, despite her depression, was not of a weakened intellect.

One may give more weight to the opinion of the psychologist who conducted the examination of the testator before she died rather than to a forensic psychiatrist who reviews the records after death and had no opportunity to conduct a face-to-face examination. However, the psychologist reached the opinion not only that the testator was depressed, but also that she had a weakened intellect and was the victim of undue influence by specific others wishing to challenge the will. Therefore, he opined that she was incompetent to write this will at that particular time. However, he did not take into account the testimony of the scrivener of the will, whose testimony indicated the strength of the mental state of the testator, which belied the opinion that she was of "weakened intellect."

It has been my experience that we should stay within the limits of our expertise, and not become adversarial in order to effect a particular conclusion in such cases. For example, we should not reach the conclusion that the person was unduly influenced, as that is a legal conclusion. We should limit our testimony to the opinion that the testator had a particular diagnosis of depression and that, as a result of that diagnosis, she was more susceptible to influence by particular others who had a close relationship with her. We do not really know whether she was unduly influenced, as that casts an aspersion on the person accused of unduly influencing her. That may have occurred, but it is not a psychiatric or psychological opinion. It is a legal conclusion.

1.14   Fees

The guidelines distinguish between retainer fees, which are ethical and appropriate, versus contingency fees, which undermine honesty and efforts to attain objectivity, and which should not be accepted [2].

Ethical questions arise beyond the issue of retainer v. contingency fees. Should psychiatrists charge first class accommodations when they travel? Should they allow themselves to be "wined and dined" by the retaining attorney? Gutheil [21] raises the question of travel expenses when one is busy enough to have more than one case away from home. How does one split the expenses and the time for the fees charged? Some psychiatrists have been known to "double bill," that is, to bill two different attorneys for the same time that was spent. That would be unethical and should be discouraged. Can a psychiatrist charge a daily fee when he travels? What about charging for overnight when one is sleeping? Should the psychiatrist charge for meals and other expenses on the road that he would normally have even if he were home?

These are questions that have not really been addressed by forensic psychiatrists traveling to examine individuals and to testify when away from home. There is also the question raised by the American Medical Association as to whether testifying in court is the practice of medicine [1]. Does a forensic medical expert need a medical license to testify in a state away from home? Some states require that one have a license in order to come to their state to conduct an examination or even to testify. Reid has conducted a survey of the various states that require licensing [22]. I do not know of any psychiatrist who has been arrested on charges of "practicing medicine without a license" for traveling to another state in order to testify. There has been one instance of a psychiatrist from a neighboring state who came in frequently to testify for the defense in criminal cases. Prosecutors became upset with him and demanded that he have a license in their state in order to come in and testify for the defense in various cases. They threatened to have him arrested for practicing medicine without a license, but he was able to obtain proper legal consultation and finally did get a license to practice medicine in the neighboring state, avoiding further legal difficulty and subsequent prosecution.

These issues of fee structure and testifying in states in which one is not licensed to practice medicine raise the question of doing harm to the forensic expert. May the expert testify in a state in which he is not licensed without being arrested for "practicing medicine without a license?" Will the expert incur harm to his or her reputation by overcharging the client for expenses on trips in which he or she travels in order to conduct examinations or to testify in different states? Most forensic psychiatrists never have to raise these questions as they are not called upon to conduct examinations away from home or to testify across the country. However, there are a handful of "super experts" who are nationally and internationally known and are often involved in very high profile cases that have national exposure. It is especially important in these cases for the expert to conduct himself or herself according to the ethical guidelines of AAPL in order to avoid bad publicity or cast aspersions on himself and, of course, also on the profession of forensic psychiatry.

1.15   Forensic v. Treatment Role

In accordance with the paper, "On wearing two hats" [23], the guidelines state that, "Psychiatrists who take on a forensic role for patients they are treating may adversely affect the therapeutic relationship with them. Treating psychiatrists should, therefore, generally avoid acting as an expert witness for their patients or performing evaluations of their patients for legal purposes" [2].

Appelbaum [24] points out the inherent dangers for the treating psychiatrist when demands are made of him to prepare a report for a legal or bureaucratic agency about information regarding his patient. One wishes to do no harm, or as little harm as possible.

Appelbaum continues questioning, "How ought a treating psychiatrist respond when a patient or the patient's lawyer requests that the psychiatrist prepare a report on the patient's suitability for custody of a child or agree to testify on the degree of emotional harm the patient suffered in an automobile accident?" [24]. Appelbaum suggests "An offer can be made to help identify another clinician to perform the forensic evaluation ... If framed properly, this response can have a powerful positive effect on the psychiatrist-patient relationship" [24].

Strasburger [23] and colleagues note it is not always possible to respond in this manner. Some agencies, such as the Social Security Administration, require statements from treating psychiatrists in adjudicating patients' disability claims. Appelbaum responds, "Failure to comply, at least at present, endangers patients' access to financial support to which they may be entitled. Moreover, in some circumstances including rural areas, there may be no other psychiatrist to whom to turn for the forensic evaluation" [24]. Appelbaum suggests discussing the problem frankly with the patient so the patient is not misled about the nature of the relationship he has with his therapist.

An example from my practice involves two of my former students who had moved to New York after training at the University of Pennsylvania. A New York attorney asked me to evaluate one of his criminal defendants, which I did and referred for treatment, giving the names of both of my former students who were practicing in New York City. The patient chose one of them for treatment, and the prosecutor chose the other (coincidentally) to conduct an examination.

The case came to trial, and the court deemed not only should I testify, but also the treating psychiatrist should testify as well. There I am in court with my two former students and now cherished colleagues, both on opposite sides. The matter was handled as pleasantly as possible, but it was important, for the outcome of the case, for the court to hear the testimony of the treating psychiatrist. Although it did have some impact on future treatment, it did not destroy the doctor-patient relationship. Treatment did continue after the hearing and did so in a positive, constructive manner.

So it is possible not to be harmful to the patient, who happens to be involved in a legal matter, for his psychiatrist to testify for him. If the testimony is conducted in a sensitive and proper manner, the doctor-patient relationship need not be negatively affected or destroyed.

1.16   Dual Role and Agency

Stone [25] critiques the question of the dual role of the forensic psychiatrist as a major concern and an ethical violation. He advocates forensic psychiatrists not working in the field because, he argues, one cannot act ethically according to the guidelines, especially if one testifies for the patient he is treating. Stone is also concerned about the dual role the psychiatrist may have when working for the prosecution in criminal cases. He notes that individuals usually see psychiatrists as helping individuals and, indeed, the forensic psychiatrist appointed by the prosecution may, in fact, be harmful to the defendant. Even discussing and disclosing his role and for whom he is working, as Appelbaum advocates, and which is part of the ethical guidelines for forensic psychiatrists, may be forgotten by the evaluee in the course of a lengthy and "seductive" examination. Thus, the evaluee may give information to the very nice and cooperative forensic psychiatrist who, in turn, may use that information against the defendant and harm him.

Stone finds Appelbaum's "Standard of Truth and Justice" more an "appealing abstraction" than a useful guide to ethical conduct in the forensic setting [25]. Stone believes that ethical behavior derived from the principles of serving truth and justice do not effectively deal with forensic psychiatry's ethical dilemma. He raises the issue of the seductive power of the forensic psychiatrist to induce inappropriate trust in an evaluee. Giving the needs of social justice primacy over helping patients, in doing no harm, Stone has argued that forensic psychiatrists lose their ethical compass.

It should be noted that the AAPL honored Professor Stone by having him lecture at their annual meeting on October 22, 1982. His remarks, entitled, "The ethical boundaries of forensic psychiatry: A view from the Ivory Tower," were published in the Bulletin of AAPL in 1984. The article was republished a quarter century later [26].

Paul Appelbaum, of whom Stone was critical, entitles his response to Stone's article, "Ethics in forensic psychiatry: Translating principles into practice" [27]. Stone has referred to Appelbaum's position as the "Standard position for ethics in forensic psychiatry." Appelbaum indicates that Stone's position has changed over 25 years when he states, "He appears to have backed away from the blanket assertion that there are no ethics principles by which the practice of forensic psychiatry can be governed, although he remains skeptical that any of the current approaches, including the Standard Position, address in practice the ethical challenges of forensic work." Appelbaum summarizes by stating that "Although the ethics challenges cannot and should not be denied, a reasonable set of ethics principles to guide forensic practice exists and, in fact, has been implicit in the work of forensic psychiatrists for many years." He believes we can "legitimately offer useful information to the courts," and that we have "a modest role, perhaps, but not one to be scorned" [27].

Griffith summarizes his position about Stone when he states, "I believe that Stone's original thoughts about ethics in forensic psychiatry, while provocative and even unnerving to his audience 25 years ago, have had a profound influence on forensic psychiatrists. The field has advanced on many fronts in the past two and a half decades" [28].

Stone's remarks at the 2007 meeting of AAPL were not published in that special edition of the Journal, so Stone published his current comments in the *Journal of Psychiatry and Law*, "Ethics in forensic psychiatry: Re-imagining the wasteland after 25 years" [29]. He summarizes by stating, "While at present there exists no uniform ethical guideline, forensic psychiatrists now have many options for moral guidance in the courtroom, and this situation is the beginning of ethical development for the profession." Basically, Stone elaborates on his epistemologic concerns about the ethics in forensic psychiatry. He refers to a recent book entitled, *Forensic Ethics and the Expert Witness*, (which he refers to as FEEW) [30] by Candilis, Weinstock, and Martinez who have been frequent contributors to the literature of ethics in psychiatry and forensic psychiatry and have done considerable research in the field. Their book, published in 2007, is a treatise on the ethical issues facing the forensic psychiatrist and expert witness. However, they do not focus on the utilization of such ethics in order to diminish the harm inherent in our work.

By contrast, this book is not a treatise on ethics in forensic psychiatry. It is about minimizing harm to those populations that are served in the legal system in administrative, civil, and criminal legal matters. Therefore, a full presentation on the Appelbaum–Stone debate is not appropriate here. However, utilizing the concepts of ethics in forensic psychiatry and how they differ from those in medicine and psychiatry generally, is helpful in understanding the purpose of this presentation.

It has always been my contention that one can get much more information from an examinee by a positive, pleasant approach than by being seen as "the enemy." When I am asked to see a defendant by the prosecution, in a criminal case, or the plaintiff by the defense attorney in a civil case, I understand that the individual may be on guard and reluctant to discuss the matter with me. I am very open with the individual, telling him who I am, whom I represent, what I will do with the information, and how it may affect him. All of this is done according to the format of the AAPL ethical guidelines [2]. However, Stone is correct in that the giving of this information can be very "seductive" and put the examinee off guard, so that he will tell me more than what he would want to or was prepared to, until he faced such a pleasant and open interviewer. Stone is also correct in that physicians are seen as helping individuals even though, in this situation, they may be harmful to the evaluee. This is one of the inherent harms built into the adversarial system in which forensic psychiatrists work on a daily basis.

Berger [31] is also concerned about ethical issues in forensic psychiatry and the matter of dual agency. He states that dual agency occurs when "a company psychiatrist owes a treatment duty to his patient—an employee of the same company—and a simultaneous obligation to the company to return the patient to work immediately." He also states there are other situations of dual agency, including "A military psychiatrist owes a treatment duty to his enlisted patient and a simultaneous duty to the military to maintain security." He further notes, "A jail psychiatrist owes a treatment duty to his inmate patient (who is awaiting his trial) and a simultaneous duty to the state to get a confession from the inmate." Also, "A state-employed psychiatrist owes a duty to the best interest of his death row patient and a simultaneous job assignment to get the execution done." He states clearly, "The two roles of the psychiatrist in these examples conflict with each other." Berger is concerned that as a therapist, the psychiatrist obtains information that can be used to relieve the patient's suffering, but the forensic psychiatrist uses his knowledge base for legal purposes. Berger concludes that "The ethical principle guiding forensic psychiatry is honesty, but a psychiatrist's honest conclusion does not always serve the best interest of the patient" [31].

Berger's examples are of people who worked for different agencies, and he stresses the job and the treatment requirements, but also the need to report to an employer about the function of the person being treated. Another example comes from a case evaluation when a judge was cited for inappropriate behavior on the bench and was told that in order to keep his job, he had to undergo treatment for several months by a psychiatrist selected by the Board of Judges. The treatment lasted for a full year. The question for the treating psychiatrist was how much he should reveal to the Board about what he learned in the course of treating the judge. Did he obtain information during treatment that would negatively affect people coming to court when the judge sat on the bench? Does the psychiatrist owe a duty, not only to his patient, but also to the community-at-large to prevent an erratic judge from retaking the bench when he may cause harm to particular individuals who come before him?

Many of us find these same questions occur when we treat individuals on probation or parole. We are asked to treat the individual primarily to keep him or her out of prison and working effectively in the community. We may also be asked to evaluate or treat people on bail awaiting trial in order to help them with their mental illness so they may be more effective at their trial, and also that they may not require hospitalization if they are found not guilty by reason of insanity or if they are found to be guilty but mentally ill and in need of treatment.

The question always arises: How much does one reveal, in the course of treatment, to the authorities, who require a regular report about the patient in treatment? This is clearly a dual role for the treating psychiatrist, who may have forensic experience. Can such a treatment be harmful to the patient if too much is revealed to the authorities? The issue here is use of good judgment in giving information that is required, but not excessive information that may prove harmful to the patient at some later time.

1.17   Deception and Forensic Practice

Bringing the matter closer to the present, Janofsky [32], in a recent article in the *Journal of AAPL* entitled, "Lies and coercion: Why psychiatrists should not participate in police and intelligence interrogations," starts by saying, "Direct or indirect participation of the psychiatrist with police, military, or intelligence personnel when interrogators use deception or psychological or physical coercion violates basic principles of ethical forensic psychiatric practice." He notes that the Appellate Court decisions have repeatedly found "that it is acceptable for police to use artifice, deception, trickery, or fraud during the course of an interrogation" [33]. He notes that psychiatrists must not engage in similar techniques, because they are unethical.

One of the examples here is the use of DNA on death row inmates to show that they could not have committed the crime for which they were convicted and sentenced to death. One case involved a man who had spent 15 years on death row after confessing to a crime that he did not commit. It was shown that the confession was made illegally through coercion and that DNA revealed his innocence and that his confession was not valid. I was asked to evaluate him to determine why he would give a confession to a crime that he did not commit. He indicated to me, on examination, that he had been coerced by the police and that he was told that if he confessed, they would let him go. At some point, he believed that to be the case rather than using logic that police would not let him go after confessing to murder. However, he was not in a logical frame of mind at the time that was offered to him.

1.18   Expert Qualifications

Finally, the guidelines refer to qualifications of the expert witness, and the commentary states, "When providing expert opinion, reports, and testimony, psychiatrists should present their qualifications accurately and precisely. As a correlate to the principle that expertise may be appropriately claimed only in areas of actual knowledge, skill, training, and experience, there are areas of special expertise, such as the evaluation of children, persons of foreign cultures, or prisoners, that may require special training or expertise" [2].

The special expertise is addressed in a book prepared by Drs. Dattilio and Sadoff about the roles and qualifications of mental health experts [34]. The book is designed to alert attorneys to the different backgrounds, education, training, and expertise of the various types of mental health experts, including psychiatrists, psychologists, social workers, and others.

Wettstein [35], in his chapter in the *Ethics Primer* of the American Psychiatric Association, discusses ethics in forensic psychiatry, and summarizes very nicely the issues of double agency and striving for objectivity and honesty. All of these are important considerations, since they go to the ultimate issue of limiting harm we do in our work in forensic psychiatry.

1.19   Ethics in Forensic Psychiatry

Weinstock has summarized an annotated bibliography on "Ethics in forensic psychiatry," in 1995 [36]. His article annotates the work of Pollack and Diamond, Appelbaum, Rosner, and Miller, and others who have worked in preparing the ethical guidelines that ultimately became the guidelines of AAPL in 2005. Furthermore, Weinstock, along with Leong and Silva [37], conducted a survey of AAPL members to determine their opinions on the inclusion of various controversial ethical issues for forensic psychiatrists. Members of AAPL appeared to appreciate the need to consider traditional Hippocratic values as at least one consideration in their functioning as forensic psychiatrists [37]. They appeared to balance their duties to an evaluee with duties to society and the legal system, and to appreciate the responsibilities of multiple agency. Support was shown for interpreting ambiguities in AAPL's current guidelines and the directions indicated by most of the survey's proposed guidelines.

The authors of the survey conclude that AAPL members clearly consider medical ethics relevant in their functioning as forensic psychiatrists. They recognize that they have multiple duties and obligations, and on occasion, they may act as double agents, or even multiple agents with multiple allegiances. The authors state, "In treatment as well as forensic situations, allegiances should be made clear. Forensic psychiatrists appear in practice to be following the balancing methods proposed by psychiatrist Edward Hundert to cope with conflicting obligations by weighing opposing values (even if not consciously), or utilizing a method similar to ethicist Baruch Brody's Model of Conflicting Appeals. In general, they do not follow any single rule or allegiance absolutely" [38].

Thus, as forensic psychiatrists, we are bound by ethical principles not only of the American Medical Association, the American Psychiatric Association, but also of the AAPL. Because there are issues of double or multiple agency built into the work of the treating psychiatrist, Appelbaum states, "If we are serious about ridding ourselves of the problem with double agency, we must begin with a code of ethics to which we adhere. When we allow therapeutic principles to creep into our thinking, we open the door to profound confusion over the psychiatrist's role" [27].

Appelbaum clearly distinguishes between treatment psychiatry and forensic psychiatry regarding ethical issues. His treatise implies that if we follow the ethical issues of forensic psychiatry, that is, respect for the individual and seeking truth and justice, we send a message to the system about our function within it. This is not to say that following the ethical guidelines of the AAPL will necessarily diminish the harm that exists within the system, but it is working in the right direction.

In commenting on Stone's thesis, Dike [39] asks, "Is ethical forensic psychiatry an oxymoron?" in which he cites a paper that I wrote in 1984, "Practical ethical problems of the forensic psychiatrist in dealing with attorneys" [40], in which I indicated that attorneys who vigorously represent the interests of their clients "may make demands on forensic psychiatrists that are either inappropriate or potentially unethical from a medical-psychiatric standpoint. They may insist that psychiatrists alter, omit, or delete information that may ultimately transform reports in favor of the attorney or patient/client." Dike notes that although my views seem to support Stone's concern that forensic psychiatrists may be cajoled by attorneys to "twist" the rules of justice in fairness to help their client, I did not see this as a reason to boycott the courts, but rather "as an indication that ethics' guidelines should be developed" [41].

Dike notes that psychiatrists, as all doctors, "take an oath to do no harm." Stone wondered whether patients may not be deceived consciously or unconsciously "and ultimately harmed, in the quest to serve justice when psychiatrists participate in the legal arena. On the other hand, the distress of cognitive dissonance that may occur in forensic psychiatrists may cause some to alter or 'twist' justice in favor of their patients (in order to do no harm)" [41].

Dike, in continuing to quote my earlier paper, reminded forensic psychiatrists that I was cognizant of the limits of individual expertise and of our profession. He notes, "If our personal biases or any information that may impair our effectiveness to the retaining attorney, the ethical forensic psychiatrist should express them to the retaining attorney especially if there is a likelihood that the biases will influence our opinion" [41].

Dike concludes, with respect to the role of the forensic psychiatrist and his place within the judicial system, as follows: "Eradicating forensic psychiatry would adversely affect the goals of achieving fairness and justice in our society. Expert opinion or testimony that leads to the hospitalization and treatment of individuals with serious mental illness in lieu of their incarceration in prison, serves not just the individual but also society at large" [41]. Dike notes that what is needed is a set of guidelines that would be pragmatic and that is tailored "to the current state of knowledge of the science of psychiatry, not to the emotional responses of those who would criticize the program" [39].

1.20 Summary

In summary, we have a very complex set of ethical guidelines and issues for the forensic psychiatrist that tend to evolve over time and with experience. We cannot use the same guidelines in forensic work as we do in treatment psychiatry. We are not there to help the individual, but to evaluate honestly and with objectivity. We can also be therapeutic in our evaluations, if we wish, in terms of helping the individual get through a very difficult evaluation that is necessary, but does not need to be destructive or damaging.

We must keep in mind that the thesis of this book is not to describe the ethical principles of medicine and psychiatry and how they differ from forensic psychiatry, but how we are guided in our work in forensic psychiatry to minimize the harm to the people we serve. Clearly, the focus is on seeking justice and respect for others. In this sense, according to Appelbaum and others who support his original and creative ideas, we can minimize harm, but not necessarily eliminate it, by adhering to accepted ethical principles.

References

1. American Medical Association (AMA) (2008) *Code of Medical Ethics: Current Opinions with Annotations, 2008–2009*. Adopted June 1957; revised June 1980. Chicago, IL.
2. American Academy of Psychiatry and the Law (AAPL) (2005) *Ethics Guidelines for the Practice of Forensic Psychiatry*. Adopted May 2005. Bloomfield, CT.
3. American Psychiatric Association (APA) (2008) *The Principles of Medical Ethics With Annotations Especially Applicable to Psychiatry*, Washington, DC.
4. Appelbaum, P.S. (1997) A theory of ethics for forensic psychiatry. *Journal of the American Academy of Psychiatry and the Law*, **25**, 233–47.
5. *Barefoot v. Estelle*, 463 US880, 903, (1983).
6. See Ref. [2], p. 4.
7. Diamond, B. (1959) The fallacy of the impartial expert. *Archives of Criminal Psychodynamics*, **3**, 221.
8. Pollack, S.D. (1974) *Psychiatry in Criminal Law*, University of Southern California Press, Los Angeles, p. 17.
9. Griffith, E.E.H. (1998) Ethics in forensic psychiatry: a cultural response to stone and appelbaum. *Journal of the American Academy of Psychiatry and Law*, **26**, 171–84.
10. See Ref. [9], p. 183.
11. Ciccone, J.R. and Clements, C.D. (2001) Commentary: Forensic psychiatry and ethics—the voyage continues. *Journal of the American Academy of Psychiatry and the Law*, **29**, 174–9.
12. Hicks, J.W. (2004) Ethnicity, race, and forensic psychiatry: are we color blind? *Journal of the American Academy of Psychiatry and the Law*, **32**, 21–33.
13. See Ref. [12], p. 23.
14. Lykken, D.T. (2000) The causes and costs of crime and a controversial cure. *Journal of Personality*, **68**, 559–614.
15. Silva, J.A. (2004) Commentary: forensic psychiatry—can its pursuit of the truth be color blind? *Journal of the American Academy of Psychiatry and the Law*, **32**, 40–2.
16. Reid, W.H. (2002) Ethics and forensic work. *Journal of Psychiatric Practice*, **8**, 380–5.
17. See Ref. [16], p. 385.
18. *Daubert v. Merrell Dow Pharmaceuticals*, 509 US 579 (1993).
19. *Kumho Tire Co. v. Carmichael*, 526 US 137, (1999).
20. *Frye v. United States*, 293 F 1013 (DC.Cir. 1923).
21. Gutheil, T.G. (1998) *The Psychiatrist as Expert Witness*, American Psychiatric Press, Washington, DC, p. 121.
22. Reid, W.H. (2000) Licensing requirements for out of state forensic examinations. *Journal of the American Academy of Psychiatry and the Law*, **28**, 433–7.
23. Strasburger, L.H., Gutheil, T.G., and Brodsky, A. (1997) On wearing two hats: role conflict in serving as both psychotherapist and expert witness. *The American Journal of Psychiatry*, **154**(4), 448–56.
24. Appelbaum, P.S. (1997) Ethics in evolution: the incompatibility of clinical and forensic functions, editorial. *The American Journal of Psychiatry*, **154**(4), 445–6.
25. Stone, A.A. (1999) The forensic psychiatrist as expert witness in malpractice cases. *Journal of the American Academy of Psychiatry and the Law*, **27**, 451–60.

26. Stone, A.A. (2008) The ethical boundaries of forensic psychiatry: a view from the Ivory Tower, reprinted. *Journal of the American Academy of Psychiatry and the Law*, **36**, 167–74.

27. Appelbaum, B.S. (2008) Ethics in forensic psychiatry: translating principles into practice. *Journal of the American Academy of Psychiatry and the Law*, **36**, 195–200.

28. Griffith, E.E.H. (2008) Stone's views of 25 years ago have now shifted incrementally. *Journal of the American Academy of Psychiatry and the Law*, **36**, 201–5.

29. Stone, A.A. with (MacCourt, D.C.) (2008) Ethics in forensic psychiatry: re-imagining the wasteland after 25 years. *Journal of Psychiatry and Law*, **36**, 617–43.

30. Candilis, P.J., Weinstock, R., and Martinez, R. (2007) *Forensic Ethics and the Expert Witness*, Springer, New York.

31. Berger, S.H. (1998) Ethics and dual agency in forensic psychiatry. *Psychiatric Times*, **15**, 6.

32. Janofsky, J. (2006) Lies and coercion: why psychiatrists should not participate in police and intelligence interrogations. *Journal of the American Academy of Psychiatry and the Law*, **34**, 472.

33. *Brown v. Mississippi*, 297 US 278, (1936).

34. Dattilio, F.M. and Sadoff, R.L. (2007) *Mental Health Experts: Roles and Qualifications for Court*, 2nd edn, PBI Press, Mechanicsburg.

35. Wettstein, R.M. (2001) Ethics and Forensic Psychiatry, in *Ethics Primer*, The American Psychiatric Association, American Psychiatric Press, Washington, DC, 65–74.

36. Weinstock, R. (1995) Ethics in forensic psychiatry—an annotated bibliography. *Bulletin of the American Academy of Psychiatry and the Law*, **23**(3), 473–82.

37. Weinstock, R., Leong, G.G., and Silva, J.A. (1991) Opinions by AAPL forensic psychiatrists on controversial ethical guidelines: a survey. *Bulletin of the American Academy of Psychiatry and Law*, **19**, 237–48.

38. See Ref. [37], p. 247.

39. Dike, C.C. (2008) Commentary: Is ethical forensic psychiatry an oxymoron? *Journal of the American Academy of Psychiatry and the Law*, **36**, 181–4.

40. Sadoff, R.L. (1984) Practical ethical problems of the forensic psychiatrist in dealing with attorneys. *Bulletin of the American Academy of Psychiatry and the Law*, **12**, 243–52.

41. See Ref. [39], p. 183.

2 Minimizing Harm: A Perspective from Forensic Psychiatry in the United Kingdom

John A. Baird

Leverndale Hospital, Glasgow, Scotland

2.1 Introduction

Forensic psychiatry practice in the United Kingdom is almost exclusively to be found within the National Health Service (NHS). The main features of the NHS are that care and treatment is free at point of delivery, it is rationed on the basis only of need. Also, healthcare professionals are salaried employees.

The risk of causing harm when practicing forensic psychiatry arises from the fact that decisions taken in forensic practice can have implications for a person which go well beyond those harmful outcomes which can occur in non-forensic psychiatric practice or in the practice of medicine generally. The opinions and decisions of forensic psychiatrists can, for example, determine significant aspects of a person's financial affairs, whether they will retain their freedom or be confined in a hospital, whether they will be convicted of a criminal offence, and whether they will be imprisoned, at which point their opinion may influence the nature and severity of the prison sentence which is imposed.

They are also expected to be able to assess the level of risk of re-offending and of the risk of harm to others. This places a major responsibility on the forensic psychiatrist which, if it goes wrong, can result in serious consequences both for the patient and those involved with him.

Ethical Issues in Forensic Psychiatry: Minimizing Harm by Robert L. Sadoff
© 2011 John Wiley & Sons, Ltd

It is probably worth clarifying that the term forensic psychiatry has a different meaning in the United Kingdom (UK) from the United States (US), and this affects in certain respects the types of harm which may follow. For what remains of this chapter I will discuss only practice in the UK, and I will leave it for an American reader to apply this to a US context.

2.2   Background

In the UK, forensic psychiatry is practiced almost exclusively within the NHS. The NHS was established in 1948, and the majority of the healthcare workforce in Britain works within its remit. A mindset of "service" is central to the work of the NHS, and this includes the forensic psychiatrist. "Service" can be clarified as an organization, such as a hospital, providing total healthcare for everyone living within a particular area. There is some private forensic practice in the UK, but it is not of a nature or extent to have a bearing on the observations and opinions which follow.

Forensic psychiatry in the UK can be divided into two groups or settings. Within the first there is the assessment, treatment, and aftercare of people who are, or may be, suffering from mental disorder and who are involved with the criminal justice system. Included in this would be care within prisons, secure hospitals—where all patients are subject to detention under the Mental Health Act—and forensic community teams where patients are usually subject to a probation or parole order. The assessment and management of the risk within this group is a crucial aspect of forensic services.

The second and complementary part of the work of a forensic psychiatrist in the UK is the role of expert witness in the criminal courts. It may come as something of a surprise to an American reader to learn that expert witness work in the civil courts in the UK is not considered to be forensic practice. There is no particular reason for this and in many respects it is somewhat illogical, but is nevertheless the current position by virtue of custom and practice. The reason may relate to the perception that civil expert witness work, unlike expert witness in the criminal courts, does not generally include an assessment of risk to others, or an assessment with the possible need for detention under mental health legislation.

Secure hospitals deal with all those patients from a particular geographical region who require to be detained under secure provision. Psychiatrists seconded to a prison will deal with all the mentally disordered offenders within this institution. Service to a geographical region, or a whole institution, is the basis of the concept of service, and forensic psychiatrists are remunerated for the service that they provide and not for the work that they do for each individual patient.

Expert witness work, however, is funded on a fee-for-service basis, but may involve patients for whom the forensic psychiatrist has an ongoing treating and clinical responsibility. The scale of payment for expert witness work is such that it only provides a small proportion of the income of most psychiatrists, whose main source of income remains their NHS salary.

The most important aspect with regard to harm minimization is a clear understanding of where and how harm may arise. Excessive risk aversion and caution, extreme use of compulsory powers under the Mental Health Act, excessive levels of physical security, and enforced medication can be as harmful as an under use of all these measures. Tragedies, such as homicides by mentally disordered people, usually arise when interventions have been inadequate, or over vigorous, when risk assessment has been incomplete or lacking in integrity and when there has been a breakdown in the communication process between the disciplines involved in patient care.

The excellent monograph by Anthony Maden (*Treating violence: A guide to risk management in mental health*) [1] discusses this whole area in some detail. From what is in effect a meta-analysis of serious untoward incidents involving the mentally disordered in England and Wales, he concludes that the two most important factors in managing a person who is mentally disordered and who presents a risk to others, is, firstly, to keep their mental illness in remission and to medicate adequately, and secondly, to respond quickly to any episodes of substance abuse.

When intervention has been inadequate, there is very often significantly increased suffering on the part of the patient and those close to them, when family have a greatly increased burden of care thrust upon them, often in circumstances where they are unable to make these difficulties known.

As with so many aspects in the practice of medicine in general, the optimal response to a particular case at a particular time requires the balancing of the advantages and disadvantages of the range of interventions which are available, and the taking of a decision which is fully informed and has accounted for all the competing aspects of the clinical problem.

2.3   Recent Developments

Over the last decade or so, there have been three developments which have contributed to improving practice in forensic psychiatry, and in particular to reducing harm. Beginning with the Ritchie report (the report of the inquiry into the care and treatment of Christopher Clunis) [2], the first development has been the importance placed on the findings of independent inquiries which are established as a matter of routine when a homicide has been committed by a person suffering from mental disorder. They are undertaken by independent panels especially appointed for the purpose, usually with a legal chair. They have access to full information of the case. They question those who were involved with the case, sometimes under oath, and they make recommendations in relation to improvements in practice which they judge to be desirable. Since 1994, these inquiry reports have led to a greater emphasis of increased management, the gathering and sharing of information, and statutory arrangements for achieving this, such as the Care Programme Approach (CPA), and Multi Agency Public Protection Arrangements (MAPPAs) [3].

In order to give practical examples of the impact of these inquiries, two recent cases will be discussed in some detail.

2.3.1 Case Example One

The report of the *Independent inquiry into the care and treatment of John Barrett* [4] described a mentally ill man who was convicted of three serious assaults in January 2002 and made the subject of a Hospital Order together with an order restricting his discharge. This option is available to courts in the UK when they deal with an offender who suffers from long-term serious mental disorder; whose offending is linked to that disorder, and whose long-term treatment and management, would best be undertaken within the mental health system. Committal is usually to a secure psychiatric hospital, and this was the case with John Barrett. By October 2003, his mental health had improved sufficiently that he was discharged with conditions by order of a Mental Health Tribunal. This is an independent body, separate from government and the judiciary, which reviews patients who are subject to detention. Mr. Barrett's mental health fluctuated thereafter and he was re-admitted on a voluntary basis on two occasions. In early September 2004, shortly after his second voluntary re-admission when he had been given time out of the hospital, he stabbed a stranger to death in a public park.

John Barrett was a man who had a long history of psychotic mental illness. He harbored a number of delusional beliefs of a paranoid nature, and the assaults which he had committed had been linked to delusional beliefs and driven by them. The inquiry panel, chaired by a solicitor and including a healthcare manager and a forensic psychiatrist, had access to all relevant documents and interviewed everyone who was involved with the case. They concluded with a report which was critical of all aspects of the patient's care, not only the individual decisions that had been taken but the management of the service which had been caring for him. They concluded "we recommend that a service improvement team, taking a national perspective, work with the Trust (the Managers) and the Forensic service, to turn around the performance of the service, to identify failings and to put in place systems and processes that are robust and effective with regular monitoring to ensure safe and effective patient care."

2.3.2 Case Example Two

The second inquiry, also published by NHS London, was the *Independent inquiry into the care and treatment of Peter Bryan and Richard Loudwell* [5]. This is a complex story and the details are extreme. Peter Bryan is a man who has psychopathic disorder and also long-term psychotic mental illness. His first homicide was in 1993. He attacked and killed a woman who was working in a shop. He was made the subject of a Hospital Order with Restriction and committed to a secure psychiatric hospital. In due course he progressed to conditional discharge and was living in the community when, in February 2004, he was charged with a second killing. On this occasion he entered a man's house, killed him, partially dismembered the body and ate portions of the man's brain. He was initially remanded to prison but his mental health deteriorated markedly, and after a few weeks in prison he was again re-admitted to a secure psychiatric hospital. Within weeks of that second admission he killed another patient, Richard Loudwell, during a short period when they were both outwith the direct supervision of nursing staff. Richard Loudwell himself was a middle-aged man who had complex mental health problems, and who had killed and sexually assaulted an elderly woman in rather bizarre circumstances. Again, the Inquiry Panel was chaired by a senior lawyer, together with a nurse manager and a consultant psychiatrist, and again recommendations were critical of many aspects of the care of these patients, including hospital management. In relation to the fatal attack on Richard Loudwell, the report concluded "No particular manager or level of management is responsible for the weaknesses we identify in relation to the attack and the issues arising from it. We see a collective failure in the organization at virtually all levels . . ."

The issues and the challenges in both these cases are very similar. In each case blame could be directed toward the clinician who took the crucial decision which allowed the homicide to occur. In one case, releasing the patient for a short period on pass and, in the other case, allowing the patient to be unsupervised while in the company of other patients. However, in each case the Inquiry team found significant shortcomings in the particular institution and service itself. To take a sporting analogy, if an ice hockey team loses by five goals to nothing, do you blame the goal-keeper who allows in the five goals, do you blame the other members of the team who did not defend adequately, do you blame the coach who is responsible for teaching the players their skills, do you blame the manager, or do you blame the chairman and the board. Tragedies of this kind and clinical decisions which, with the benefit of hindsight, were wrong, may be most likely to occur in organizations which are themselves dysfunctional at all levels.

Individual institutions, hospitals, and trusts also hold internal Critical Incident Reviews (CIRs) and Serious Untoward Incident Investigations (SUIIs) which are less formal than the independent inquiry, but probably do not have the opportunity for detachment and objectivity which is necessary to reveal underlying shortcomings as independent inquiries are able to do.

The second development has been the recent changes in procedures which were introduced in order to try to ensure fairness in decision making. The changes affected many aspects of society and arose from the UK becoming a signatory of the European Convention on Human Rights. In relation to mental health procedures, an independent authority—the Mental Health Tribunal—was established, with the power to detain patients, to review their detention and to order their release if their detention is not justified. Their powers extend to those patients who have been involved with serious offending and who have been committed to a hospital by a criminal court, subject not only to an order in terms of the Mental Health Act, but to an order restricting their discharge [6]. The legislation here is complex, but for present purposes it is only important to emphasize that before Human Rights legislation came into force in 1999, decisions in relation to restricted patients were taken by politicians, namely the Home Secretary.

This compromised independence and allowed politicians to take decisions about patients while influenced by wider political considerations, rather than on the merits of the individual case. There was also a view that politicians were slow to take decisions and were excessively cautious. Although detailed research has not yet been possible during the time that Mental Health Tribunals have been in force, the consequences of giving the decision to an independent body have been interesting and at times unexpected. The tribunals may, in certain circumstances, be no less cautious than were the politicians. As the decisions are taken by different groups of three individuals, there is the potential, on occasion, for unexpected decisions to be reached. There can be no doubt, however, that since coming into existence, these independent tribunals have been able to take courageous and radical decisions in circumstances when this was required, and have managed to cut through the bureaucracy which can be associated with certain complex cases. New systems require time to become established but it can already be acknowledged that they represent a very considerable improvement on what went before.

The third development, over the last decade, has been the importance attached to the field of risk assessment. Previously, assessment of risk was largely unstructured and relied upon what has been termed the "charismatic authority" of the assessing psychiatrist (see Risk for Sexual Violence Protocol Manuel) [7]. Techniques have since developed into the numerical-based actuarial methods now practiced, and more recently, into a structured clinical judgment approach, where information is gathered systematically but then evaluated by a trained professional. Risk assessment instruments are now also beginning to be considered, where some emphasis can be placed on the positive factors of the individual.

Harm reduction is an issue which has had considerable prominence in the UK over the last 15 years. The better the service, the organization and the practice, the less the risk of harm is likely to be. As in any complex professional task, clinical excellence is achieved by working closely with colleagues, respecting the judgment of others and having the confidence to challenge when the need arises. This professional environment toward which we are all working will achieve the best possible outcome in these areas of high risk. "Healthy" institutions, together with patient safety and public safety, is probably a shared aspiration both in the UK and the US and on this final point there this is likely to be no difference between the two sides of the Atlantic.

References

1. Maden, A. (2007) *Treating Violence: A guide to risk management in mental health*, Oxford University Press.
2. Ritchie, J., Dick, D., and Lingham, R. (1994) *The Report of the Inquiry into the care and treatment of Christopher Clunis*, HMSO, London.
3. Royal College of Psychiatrists (2005) *Psychiatrists and Multi-Agency Public Protection Arrangements: Guidelines on Representation, Participation, Confidentiality and Information Exchange*, Author, London.
4. NHS London (2006) *Report of the Independent Inquiry into the care and treatment of John Barrett*, Author.

5. NHS London (2009) *Independent Inquiry into the care and treatment of Peter Bryan and Richard Loudwell*, Author.

6. Millan Committee (2001) Report on the Review of the Mental Health (Scotland) Act 1984 SE/2001/56.

7. Hart, S.D., Kropp, P.R., Laws, D.R. *et al.* (2003) The Risk for Sexual Violence Protocol (RSVP): Structured Professional Guidelines for Assessing Risk of Sexual Violence, Mental Health, Law and Policy Institute, Simon Fraser University, Burnaby.

3 Mental Health and Human Rights in Forensic Psychiatry in the European Union

Emanuele Valenti

European University of Madrid, Madrid, Spain

Luis Fernando Barrios Flores

Department of State Legal Studies, University of Alicante, Alicante, Spain

3.1 Introduction

Mental health has been a debated topic in most of the Western European States since the 1980s. In order to understand the reasons for this interest, it is necessary to reflect on the cultural and political unification processes amongst the European States since the first half of the twentieth century, as a consequence of post-World War II events.

The unification of Europe is a very slow process, which began before the actual European Union (EU) was founded. It responds to the need of every European State to reach common political, economic, social, and cultural objectives.

One of the most important events characterizing the process of transition to the EU was the signing of the *Convention for the Protection of Human Rights and Fundamental Freedoms* by the Council of Europe Member States in 1950. From then on, the topic of human rights became the inspiring principle in the construction of the European Community (EC), and following on the institutional apparatus that constitutes the Union.

Ethical Issues in Forensic Psychiatry: Minimizing Harm   by Robert L. Sadoff
© 2011 John Wiley & Sons, Ltd

The Council of Europe's first recommendation on mental health was adopted in 1977, after which the Council's activity on this topic progressively increased throughout the 1980s and 1990s. It stimulated a debate amongst civilian society, as represented by user associations, and professionals. This enriched and increased the States' legislative activity at a national level, and produced a group of reforms of health policy, which led to a process of modernization of the majority of the Community's mental health services.

This transformation was developed in two main stages: in the first phase the *welfare state* was created by means of extending social security to all citizens. This era also saw the diffusion of new contributions to mental health care, including private psychiatry, the advent of psychoactive medications and the creation of out-patient care centers in psychiatric hospitals. The second phase began in the 1970s, and is marked by a long-term action plan drafted by the World Health Organization (WHO) Regional Office for Europe, which started a de-institutionalizing process of mental health. Since then it has been developed in mental health institutes and has built up community-based mental health care.

The core of this process has consisted in a structural transformation of the relations between the care providers and the community. Historically, providers were divided between the community and the mental hospital, maintaining a give-and-take relationship that could be described as a "vertical" structure. Changes have led to a different "horizontal" structure, where the system has been formed by—in addition to the family—psychiatrists and a care team consisting of psychologists, social workers, some occupational therapists, and other specific roles [1].

Contemporary mental health care is a synthesis between an integrated system of vertical care and a systematic horizontal care. The process of extending community-based care continues across Europe, indicating a trend toward integrating mental health care in primary medicine. This integration is the result of a new perspective, focused on overcoming the traditional dichotomy between the centralized role of the mental hospital on one hand and the importance of treatment and care in the community setting on the other.

The new tendency in the EU is to consider these two perspectives as mutually exclusive, and to favor a new philosophy of mental health in which balanced care includes both community-based and hospital-based care. The basic principles of this new form of community psychiatry are extended along the following guidelines: (i) the de-institutionalization process and closure of old mental hospitals; (ii) the development of alternative community services and programs; and (iii) the integration of basic health services with social and community services [2].

The political context of mental health reform is very different in each geographical area, and its outcome is only at the regional level. For this reason the process of psychiatric reform in Europe is a pending issue. In Central and Eastern Europe the collapse of centralized command economies had a strong impact upon the mental health of the population and financial constraints have hampered reforms; de-institutionalization may be seen as an opportunity to reduce costs, but insufficient funds can be transferred to alternative community-based care because of budgetary constraints [3].

The primary objective of the EU States currently is to promote a harmonization of the different national legislations on mental health, favoring a central health policy that will reduce inequalities amongst the Member States [4].

Since 2002, research programs have been set up to identify the differences between the various national mental health services in the EU, with the aim of developing a reform program of equal efficiency in all of the Community countries.

In this chapter, we will present the aspects of European mental health reform that affect forensic psychiatry in relation to legal frameworks, routine procedures, and ethical issues.

3.2 Forensic Psychiatry in the European Union

The EU is comprised of 27 Member States, although the Council of Europe plans to extend this to 45 States including some countries of Eastern Europe and Turkey. This reality makes it necessary to consider the creation of tools that will allow a way to deal with the mobility of citizens from very diverse countries and cultures [5].

Another aspect that is very present in forensic psychiatry today is the task of harmonizing mental health legislation. Research in this area aims to respond to the demands raised in attempting to harmonize the very different judicial systems that are applied with great variety at regional and national level in each Member State.

In the EU, two different judicial traditions coexist: Roman law and common law. The first constitutes the basis for the majority of the continental countries and is inspired by the Greco-Roman tradition. It underwent a long development during the Middle Ages in Central Europe, and extended over all of Europe as a result of the French Revolution. The main characteristic of Roman law is the prescriptive nature of its rules. The laws establish what a crime is and what is legal, and they define the procedures and the punishments that the judges may establish with ample discretionary authority. The interpretation of the judicial codes is limited and represents an important element in all judgments, while jurisprudence plays a minor role. The consequence of such a system affects the time needed to define reform processes, and the flexibility of the judicial system, which is poor when the time comes to adapting the rules to specific situations.

The country which most closely follows the Roman law model is Germany. The Mediterranean countries have simpler systems which leave more discretional power to the judges than other countries.

France, Belgium, and Holland all have a more flexible system that is capable of adapting to individual cases. The Scandinavian countries leave a lot of room for civil law and have more complete judicial systems. In relation to forensic psychiatry, Roman law assigns a very important role to the psychological component of the crime and to criminal responsibility. For this reason, an individual who suffers a mental disorder may not bear the full weight of responsibility, as with children, and is thus able to avoid criminal sanctions.

Common law constitutes the judicial foundation for all those European countries with an Anglo-Saxon tradition. The administration of justice is less prescriptive than in Roman law. Its pragmatic focus puts more emphasis on behavior than on the psychological aspect, and gives less relevance to the role of criminal responsibility. The power of the judge is concentrated on determining whether or not the criminal act was committed. The consequences of this are reflected in the existence of a more flexible judicial system and proceedings which are more adaptable to the event's circumstances [6].

This chapter presents some of the areas, of particular relevance to the field of forensic psychiatry, which are undergoing mental health reforms. These reforms will in turn directly affect health professionals, lawyers, users, and politicians.

All the Member States have specific laws, codes, and other legal tools to regulate judicial proceedings that involve patients with mental disorders who have been arrested. The forensic legislation in most countries depends on the criminal code and mental health laws. In some countries national legislation is integrated with regional legislation that is in force only in certain areas of the State [7].

The reason for these variations is explained by the different elements that come into play in the field of forensics. Some States do not have a single forensic code, while others have recently reformed their laws on mental health and have demanded evidence of these reforms in the practice of forensics.

The plurality of systems is also reflected in the terminology used in forensic psychiatry, which varies according to the codes of each country. Most of these are influenced by the *DSM-IV*[1] or *ICD-10*[2]. Many of the terms used in the codes are very descriptive and are not used in a precise manner, assuming different meanings in each State of the Union. Definitions of serious illnesses such as schizophrenia are sometimes generically defined simply as a "psychotic state". The emotional disorders or organic pathologies may be considered differently depending on the judges, psychiatrists, courts, or other authorities involved in a trial. Many mental disorders such as drug addictions, personality disorders, or paraphilias may not be subject to forensic legislation because they are criminally relevant only in a few countries. Likewise, disorders related to alcohol lack defined guidelines, thus the criminal consequences of crimes committed while under the influence of alcohol may be very different depending on the country and the individual situation.

In all of the EU Member States, those arrested with mental disorders can be admitted to specialized institutions such as forensic hospitals, general psychiatric hospitals, psychiatric wards in general hospitals, prisons, or therapeutic communities [5].

One very controversial aspect is the sequence of forensic treatment and judicial sentencing. Only in seven countries (Austria, Belgium, Germany, Italy, The Netherlands, Portugal, and Spain) is there specific legislation which establishes the provisional sequence for the two events. In the other States, the judge adopts

---

[1] *Diagnostic and Statistical Manual of Mental Disorders*, Fourth edition, published by the American Psychiatric Association.
[2] *International Statistical Classification of Diseases and Related Health Problems*, 10th Revision, published by the World Health Organization.

an individualized measure, according to the circumstances. Although this aspect may raise doubts for security reasons, there are clinical arguments that support a flexible individual regulation, specific to the severity of the pathology and the patient's health condition. In the cases where there is a sentence and judicial order for treatment, many States subtract the period of treatment from the overall sentence set by the judge. Flexible proceedings are adopted in cases when there is not a clear diagnosis: the defendant has committed another crime, due to the patient's health, or for public safety [8]. In Europe, forensic psychiatry is considered a medical specialty that is part of psychiatry. It has a very important role because it can influence many of the related consequences of a sentencing, treatment, or of a detainee being admitted. The assessment of a defendant by a forensic psychiatrist represents the meeting point between mental health services and the judicial system, such that it is necessary to establish clear rules and procedures that define the role of each. In two-thirds of the Member States, the intervention of a forensic psychiatrist is legally required for all detainees who suffer a mental disorder [9]. In the countries where there is not a specific legal regulation, psychiatrists from the public health department are in charge of making forensic assessments. The forensic assessments can be a requirement in case of medical-legal problems, especially in relation to cases in which the patient's capacity of control could lead to a repeat of the crime. The exceptions are in Denmark and the United Kingdom where this task is demanded of a psychiatric hospital [10].

With respect to the education of forensic psychiatrists, no requirement exists that establishes a certain level of specific experience or practical training to be able to practice this profession. Having a degree in psychiatry is sufficient. In some States, forensic studies are part of the university curriculum in the medical faculty. Only Finland requires six years of training in the field of forensics apart from clinical activities such as psychiatry, while in the United Kingdom and Germany, forensics studies last for three years, as a postgraduate program after obtaining a degree in psychiatry. Portugal requires only six months of studies. The EU's legal regulations do not establish a specific course of study for forensic psychiatry. This has consequences on the quality of these degrees, which generally are varied and insufficient. In the opinion of many forensic psychiatrists, it is necessary to define a mandatory curriculum that can guarantee equality of service for all mentally ill citizens undergoing criminal proceedings.

3.3 Human Rights, Mental Health, and Forensic Psychiatry in Europe

What we are proposing is a global vision of the European system of guarantees for people suffering from mental disorders. The national responses to the recognition of the Council of Europe's recommendations, and the statements issued by the European Court of Human Rights suffer from important deficiencies and often are not recognized by the courts of some States. Notwithstanding, they have a great deal of influence on new reforms in the mental health systems in the majority of the countries of the Union, and are a reference for all the States that were recently inducted into the EU.

Movements for the humanization of assistance for the mentally ill have been emerging in Europe for the past 200 years. Although it is fair to recognize their existence, they were fundamentally based on religious criteria. The Tuke family in the York Retreat applied the principle of non-restraint [11] which was carried on by Robert G. Hill and John Conolly, and spread throughout Europe [12]. On the continent itself, Colombier and Doublet were the authors of *Gouverner les Insensés* [13], Philippe Pinel wrote *Traité Médico-philosophique sur l'Aliénation mentale* [14] and was involved in the effort to remove the mentally ill from their chains. However, it is also fair to recognize that such an initiative was inspired by the humanitarian treatment that Poussin and his wife had previously applied to mental patients, which appealed to Pinel intensely.

In the nineteenth century there was also an articulated response on the guarantees for psychiatric admissions. Incomprehensibly, the French Civil Code of March 21, 1804, evaded regulating psychiatric internments, something regarded as unavoidable by the other European Codes. To satisfy such a gap, the French law on the insane was passed on June 30, 1838, which was followed by different regulations in other countries.

Nevertheless, the systematic protection of the rights of the mentally ill in Europe really only progressed during the twentieth century, mostly through the work of the Council of Europe. Although other organizations made some effort in this area, for example, the EU and the WHO Regional Office for Europe, the Council was responsible for the most extensive and intensive labor in this field as emphasized above.

3.4   The Council of Europe

Founded in London in 1949, today 47 States comprise the Council of Europe. It provides a framework of reference of rules and a widespread regime of guarantees on the subject of human rights in general, and with respect to the protection of these rights specifically in the scope of care of mental patients.

3.4.1   The Recommendations of the Council of Europe

By way of recommendations, the Consultative Assembly take their conclusions to the Committee of Ministers, and from the Committee of Ministers these are taken to the governments of the Member States. In the past few decades, the following recommendations have been approved with regard to mental health and the protection of the mentally ill:

- Rec. 818 (1977), relating to the situation of the mentally ill (Parliamentary Assembly, 12th meeting, October 8, 1977).
- Rec. No. R (80) 4, regarding the patient as an active participant in their own treatment (Committee of Ministers, 318th meeting, April 30, 1980).

- Rec. No. R (83) 2, on the legal protection for people suffering mental illnesses and admitted as involuntary patients (Committee of Ministers, 356th meeting February 22, 1983).
- Rec. No. R (87) 3, on European penitentiary rules (Committee of Ministers, 404th meeting, December 12, 1987.
- Rec. No. R (91) 15, on European cooperation with respect to epidemiological studies in the field of mental health (Committee of Ministers, 463rd meeting, October 11, 1991).
- Rec. 1185 (1992), on rehabilitation policies for disabled persons (Parliamentary Assembly, 6th meeting, May 7, 1992).
- Rec. No. R (92) 6, on a coherent policy with respect to the integration of handicapped persons (Committee of Ministers, 474th meeting, April 9, 1992).
- Rec. 1235 (1994), regarding psychiatry and human rights (Parliamentary Assembly, 10th meeting, April 12, 1994).
- Rec. No. R (98) 7, concerning ethical and organizational aspects of health care in the penitentiary setting (Committee of Ministers, 627th meeting, April 8, 1998).
- Rec. (2004) 10, relates to the protection of human rights and the dignity of persons suffering from mental illnesses (Committee of Ministers, 896th meeting, September 22, 2004).
- Rec. (2006) 2, on European Prison Rules (Committee of Ministers, 952nd meeting, January 11, 2006).
- Rec. (2009) 3, on a follow-up of the protection of human rights and the dignity of persons suffering from mental illnesses (Committee of Ministers, 1057th meeting, May 20, 2009).

Focusing on the last few citations, which compile, update, and incorporate significant modifications to earlier recommendations, Rec. (2004) 10 is very detailed and without a doubt constitutes the main reference with respect to the protection of mental patients' rights in Europe. It is devoted to anti-discriminatory principles (Art. 3), conservation of the practice of mental patients' civil rights and policies (Art. 4), minimal restrictions (Art. 8), and equipping psychiatric establishments' living conditions to general welfare standards (Art. 9).

Similar criteria are established for involuntary detention and treatment (Art. 17–18): (i) the person must be suffering from a mental disorder, (ii) their behavior must present a serious risk to themselves or others, (iii) there must not be any less restrictive means of providing appropriate care available, and (iv) the opinion of the afflicted person must be taken into consideration.

According to Rec. (2004) 10, involuntary treatment must: (i) respond to specific signs or symptoms, (ii) be proportionate to their health condition, (iii) have therapeutic purpose, (iv) be administered by qualified staff, (v) be part of a written plan, (vi) be substituted as quickly as possible by voluntary treatment, (vii) have consulted—whenever possible—with the concerned person, and (viii) be periodically reevaluated (Art. 12, 17(iii), and 19).

Regarding involuntary admissions (Art. 20–25): (i) the decision must be made by a court or competent request (this distinction is motivated by the heterogeneity of guarantee systems in the various European countries), taking into consideration the patient's opinion and respecting the legally required proceedings, (ii) documentation must be submitted, establishing the maximum time period for reevaluations, without jeopardizing the patient's right to request the same and utilize the corresponding resources, (iii) must be based on a medical report, (iv) the patient's representative and those close to the patient must be informed and consulted with, (v) must end if the placement criteria are not met, (vi) the patient's right to know why the decision was made for detention, the criteria for the stay's duration, and the available resources, such as the right to communicate with their lawyer or representative without unreasonable visitation limits must be guaranteed, and (vii) a rigorous system of resources must be described. As far as urgent admissions are concerned, it is recommended that these should only be on a short-term basis, and if an admission is to be extended, the decision must be made by a court or other competent request. Rec. (2004) 10 even provides for the possibility, although as an exception and only for the minimum amount of time necessary, for an evaluation to "determine if [the concerned person] is suffering from a mental disorder which represents a real risk of serious injury to their health or to the health of others." In such a case the requirements are that: (i) the behavior suggests grounds for the existence of such a disorder, (ii) their condition allows the supposition of said risk, (iii) no other less restrictive means of evaluating their condition exist, and (iv) the concerned person's opinion will be taken into consideration (Art. 17.2).

The use of other coercive methods, such as isolation and restraints, demands medical supervision, observance of the principle of minimal restriction, submission of documentation, and continuous follow-up (Art. 27). This aspect is regulated very little, if at all in national legislations. It needs urgent attention in order to apply some basic principles that guarantee rights, as well as for the mental patient's own care.

Treatments that produce irreversible physical effects or that suppose a significant intrusion should be evaluated from an ethical standpoint. They should be performed according to clinical protocols and the treatment must be properly documented, recommending that they not take place in the context of an involuntary placement (Art. 28).

Article 37 of Rec. (2004) 10 establishes a set of control mechanisms: visits and inspections in psychiatric establishments, including without prior notice; official institution records; verification of compliance with professional standards; evaluation of communication restrictions, or an independent investigation in case of a death in these establishments.

With respect to mental patients admitted to penitentiary establishments, Rec. (2004) 10 indicates that no discrimination is tolerated; they should receive the appropriate therapeutic methods available, and an independent system of control for treatment and care (Art. 35).

Recommendation (2006) 2 is exclusively dedicated to the latter topic, the European Penitentiary Rules. These advocate coordination between penitentiary health care and the national health care system of each State (40.1 and 2). They also establish: the need to detect mental suffering (40.4), the institution or special section's resources for the observation and treatment of detainees of this type (47.1), and pay special attention to suicide prevention (47.2).

Recommendation (2009) 3 was recently approved, and takes Rec. (2004) 10 as its starting point. It serves as a reminder that in the first place is the need to assure that there is no discrimination against the mental patient, even allowing the use of affirmative action so that persons with mental disorders may take part in social activities. It invites the Member States to adopt, on one hand, legal measures to avoid discrimination, and, on the other hand, administrative measures that make the socio-labor integration of the mentally handicapped possible. It also urges the development of campaigns against stigmatization and for professional training, especially for police and teachers (Principle 1). With respect to civil and political rights, it proposes the most complete guarantees possible of upholding these rights on behalf of persons suffering from mental disorders. It creates control and defense mechanisms, and promotes the participation of this group of citizens, including access to public service, as well as the most scrupulous respect for the confidentiality of data and privacy (Principle 2). The objective of Principle 3 is the promotion of health. There is the necessity to implement instruments and programs to protect vulnerable people (Principle 4): the persecution of those responsible for potential abuses in the prison environment; the provision of training so that attending staff can detect abuses; from a welfare point, the provision of resources to entities that guarantee assistance, and the protection of this group of patients in the practice of biomedical research. The quality of living conditions, welfare services and treatments must be promoted (Principle 5). It places special importance on the establishment of standards of quality and verification of their practical application. This includes taking into account the singular importance that such effect has on the users' participation. Recommendation (2009) 3 reiterates the necessity of applying methods that are the least restrictive possible of personal freedom in the establishments and other welfare services (Principle 6). As indicated by its title, this Recommendation invites the States to establish adequate legal frameworks to protect persons suffering from mental disorders, especially with regard to involuntary treatment and internments (Principle 7). Finally, Principle 8 tackles a subject that historically has tended to be overlooked: the rights and care of the friends and relatives of mental patients.

3.4.2 The European Convention on Human Rights

The *Convention for the Protection of Human Rights and Fundamental Freedoms* was approved on November 4, 1950, and entered into force on September 3, 1953. Its articulations contain various precepts that influence mental health, but which are not applicable by law. However, the entire recommendation of this Convention can be applied in the field of mental health:

- Article 3. "No one shall be subjected to torture or to inhuman or degrading punishment or treatment."

- Article 5.1. "Everyone has the right to liberty and security of person. No one shall be deprived of his liberty save in the following cases and in accordance with a procedure prescribed by law . . ."
- Article 5.1.(e). "the lawful detention of persons for the prevention of the spreading of infectious diseases, of persons of unsound mind, alcoholics or drug addicts or vagrants;"
- Article 5.4. "Everyone who is deprived of his liberty by arrest or detention shall be entitled to take proceedings by which the lawfulness of his detention shall be decided speedily by a court and his release ordered if the detention is not lawful."
- Article 5.5. "Everyone who has been the victim of arrest or detention in contravention of the provisions of this Article shall have an enforceable right to compensation."
- Article 6.1. " . . . everyone is entitled to a fair and public hearing within a reasonable time by an independent and impartial tribunal established by law . . ."
- Article 8.1. "Everyone has the right to respect for his private and family life, his home and his correspondence."

The interest in these rules is doubled, not only because their ratification supposes a link between the States, but also because they have given way for the elaboration of an interesting law of precedence by the overseeing body in the Convention, the European Court of Human Rights, as foreseen in Article 19(b), and developed in Articles 38–56 of the Convention.

3.4.3   Jurisprudence of the European Court of Human Rights

On September 18, 1959, the European Court of Human Rights was created in Strasbourg, within the framework of the Convention, with the mission to oversee the integrity of the compromises adopted by the agreeing States. On November 1, 1998, according to the provisions of Protocol No. 11 to the Convention, the European Court of Human Rights was restructured and established as a single and permanent full-time Court.

The European Court of Human Rights' conclusions form a legal doctrine, which is an inevitable reference for the protection of mental patients in Europe, especially with regard to the guarantees and conditions of psychiatric internment. The following cases are the main resolutions referencing this topic: *Winterwerp v. The Netherlands*, 24 October 1979; *X v. United Kingdom*, 5 November 1981; *Luberti v. Italy*, 23 February 1984; *Ashingdane v. United Kingdom*, 28 May 1985; *Nielsen v. Denmark*, 28 November 1988; *Van der Leer v. The Netherlands*, 21 February 1990; *E. v. Norway*, 29 August 1990; *Wassink v. The Netherlands*, 27 September 1990; *Koendjbiharie v. The Netherlands*, 25 October 1990; *Keus v. The Netherlands*, 25 October 1990; *Megyeri v. Germany*, 12 May 1992; *Herczegfalvy v. Austria*, 24 September 1992; *Silva Rocha v. Portugal*, 15 November 1996; *Eriksen v. Norway*, 27 May 1997; *Johnson v. United Kingdom*, 24 October 1997; *Aerts v. Belgium*, 30 July 1998; *Erkalo v. The Netherlands*, 2 September 1998; *Varbanov v. Bulgaria*,

5 October 2000; *D.N. v. Switzerland*, 29 March 2001; *Keenan v. United Kingdom*, 3 April 2001; *Rutten v. The Netherlands*, 24 July 2001; *Magalhaes Pedreira v. Portugal*, 26 February 2002; *H.M. v. Switzerland*, 26 February 2002; *Paul & Audrey Edwards v. United Kingdom*, 14 March 2002; *Lutz v. France (1)*, 26 March 2002; *L.R. v. France*, 27 June 2002; *Nouhaud et al. v. France*, 9 July 2002; *Hutchison Reid v. United Kingdom*, 20 February 2003; *Herz v. Germany*, 12 June 2003; *Lutz v. France (2)*, 17 June 2003; *Tracik v. Slovakia*, 14 October 2003; *Rakevich v. Russia*, 28 October 2003; *Worwa v. Poland*, 27 November 2003; *Morsink v. The Netherlands*, 11 April 2004; *M.R.L. & M.-J.D. v. France*, 19 May 2004; *Tam v. Slovakia*, 22 June 2004; *H.L. v. United Kingdom*, 5 October 2004; *Kolanis v. United Kingdom*, 21 June 2005; *Storck v. Germany*, 16 June 2005.

In the resolutions of these cases, the following issues were considered to be the most relevant. Starting with the indispensable requirements for involuntary internment (*Winterwerp v. Holland*, § 39), requirements which are reiterated in *X v. United Kingdom*, § 40; *Ashingdane v. United Kingdom*, § 37; *Johnson v. United Kingdom*, § 60; *M.R.L. & M.-J.D. v. France*, § 115, among other resolutions:

1. The prior verification of the person's mental condition by means of a medical evaluation is "not only possible, but is indispensable" to be able to proceed to a non-urgent detention (*Varbanov v. Bulgaria*, § 48). By not conducting such a verification, the detention will have a different functionality, for example, administrative, thus violating Article 5.1 of the European Convention on Human Rights (*M.R.L. & M.-J.D. v. France*, §§ 117, 120, and 128). Exceptions to this requirement are those of supposed urgency which demand a quick judicial response (*Herz v. Germany*, § 46). A "provisional detention" is also allowed [sic], based on Article 5.1.(c) of the European Convention of Human Rights, when "probable cause exists to prevent the commission of a criminal offense" (*Eriksen v. Norway*, § 86).
2. A mental disorder of such a nature and to such an extent that it justifies internment (*Winterwerp v. The Netherlands*, § 39).
3. The involuntary internment must not be prolonged to exceed said disorder, although difficulties in risk assessment require the allowance of certain flexibility for the decisive authorities (*Johnson v. United Kingdom*, §§ 61 and 63).

In order for a decision for detention to not violate Article 5.4 of the European Convention of Human Rights, it must come from a body with distinctive features of a "court" possessing the characteristics of a "court" (*Winterwerp v. The Netherlands*, § 67). For the detention to be "lawful", extracts in Article 5.1.(e) of the European Convention on Human Rights, it should be executed in a "hospital, clinic, or other appropriate establishment which has been habilitated for that purpose" (*Ashingdane v. United Kingdom*, § 44; in the same context, *Aerts v. Belgium*, § 46.). In *Aerts v. Belgium*, the psychiatric wing of a prison is not considered appropriate due to the fact that the mentally unsound "do not receive medical attention nor are they in a therapeutic setting" (§ 49), although a violation of Article 3 of the Convention was not noted. A prolonged stay in such a facility may present a notable risk of aggravating the patient's mental health condition, although it was not believed to be what happened in this particular case (§§ 65–66).

"The patient's right to adequate treatment for their condition cannot be deduced from Article 5.1.(e) of the European Convention on Human Rights" (*Winterwerp v. The Netherlands*, § 51). But this must be duly interpreted since, at its core, what the European Court of Human Rights means to express is that the European Convention on Human Rights has content referring to formal liberties, but not to provisional rights, with regard to treatment.

Detention and deprivation are different measures; for that reason, any restriction of the capacity to administer one's own affairs must be made with the guarantees of Article 6.1 of the European Convention of Human Rights (*Winterwerp v. The Netherlands*, § 75).

The chapter of guarantees of the European Convention of Human Rights indicates that Article 5.1.(a) is also applicable to psychiatric internment for criminal purposes, although in these cases the implementation of confinement is superimposed (a) and (e) of the mentioned Article 5.1. (*X v. United Kingdom* § 39; also in *Johnson v. United Kingdom*, § 58). Besides that, as indicated in *Eriksen v. Norway* § 76, a detention may be justified depending on the circumstances, by more than one section of said precept. Regarding the scope of subjectivity, upon review "the guarantee ensures that it also applies to minors" (*Nielsen v. Denmark*, § 58); although in this case it was not the application of the guarantee, by executing the detention by use of parental authority and not by decision of the State (§§ 63–64).

Among the guarantees of jurisprudence of the European Court of Human Rights considered to be indispensable are:

- The notification of the motives for detention (as shown in case *Van der Leer v. The Netherlands*), despite the use of certain terms of criminal connotation in Article 5.2 of the European Convention of Human Rights (§ 27), indicate that there is no doubt of its application to the present material (§ 29). However, as it is logical, the lack of notification of the decision to extend an internment is justified in the case of the patient being incoherent at the time the decision is made (*Keus v. The Netherlands*, § 22).
- "An attorney's assistance in subsequent proceedings related to the continuation, suspension, or termination of detention" (*Megyeri v. Germany*, § 23); which also occurred in *Aerts v. Belgium*, where a violation of Article 6.1 of the European Convention of Human Rights was noted, by not acknowledging the right to legal assistance in an appeal before the Court of Cassation of Belgium, since the actual matter in issue was not just the mere topic of inter-institutional transfer, but was actually the "lawfulness of the deprivation of liberty" (§ 59).

The guarantees as established by the national legislation must likewise be taken into account. For this reason, the failure to comply with the extension of detention time periods, as in *Erkalo v. The Netherlands*, is considered to be a violation of Article 5.1 of the European Convention of Human Rights. In *Van der Leer v. The Netherlands*, the lack of a legally required hearing falls into the same category

(§ 23). The same thing happened with *Wassink v. The Netherlands*, due to the absence of a court clerk during the hearing, as required by Dutch legislation (§ 27).

All those who are involuntarily detained, must have the right to legally appeal the grounds for their detention. With respect to fact that it must be understood as a court, several of the Convention's articles make use of said purpose, indicating that it must be a body which maintains independence with regards to the execution, to the parties and respects the guarantees of a judicial proceeding (*De Wilde, Ooms, & Versyp v. The Netherlands*, sentencing by the European Court of Human Rights, June 18, 1971, § 78), which does not necessarily need to be "a conventional type of jurisdiction" (*X v. United Kingdom*, § 3). Besides this, it is necessary that the proceedings "be of a judicial character and provide the charged individual corresponding guarantees as to the nature of the deprivation of their liberty" (*De Wilde*, § 76). Therefore, in *X v. United Kingdom* the violation of Article 5.4 of the European Convention of Human Rights was noted due to the fact that the *Mental Health Review Tribunals* (from the *Mental Health Act* of 1959 and not the subsequent 1983 Act) could periodically evaluate the situation of the detainee, but "lacked competence to decide 'about the lawfulness of the detention' and to order their freedom would have been considered illegal" (*X v. United Kingdom*, § 61). A *habeas corpus* is not enough to fully understand an effective judicial protection, because its limited control is insufficient for the hypothesis of a prolonged detention (*idem*, § 58).

The "court" must be impartial with respect to other bodies, but also internally, subjectively, which "is presumed, until proven otherwise", as well as objectively, given the importance that "simple appearances" have, and the "confidence that the courts of a democratic society should be inspiring as justiciable, especially to the parties in litigation" (*D.N. v. Switzerland*, §§ 44–46). For this reason it is unacceptable that someone who acts as a legal expert also forms part of the court (*idem*, § 55).

In several declarations, the European Court of Human Rights has stated the interpretation of Article 5.4 of the European Convention on Human Rights, as it relates to the speediness of the "judicial" body's response, so that the lawfulness of the detention may be determined. The following are considered as being unjustified: 15 months or 2 years (*Herczegfalvy v. Austria*, §§ 77–78), 18 months and 10 days (*Luberti v. Italy*, § 37), 5 months (*Van der Leer v. The Netherlands*, § 36), 4 months (*Koendjbiharie v. The Netherlands*, § 29), or 5 weeks (*E. v. Norway*, §§ 65–66). In *Varbanov v. Bulgaria* the same precept was noted to have been violated by the Bulgarian legislation by not allowing for a rapid appeal (§§ 60–61).

Transportation between psychiatric institutions was addressed in *Ashingdane v. United Kingdom*. The difficulties presented by a transfer between a high-security institution and an ordinary institution were brought before the court to declare that, although the latter is more liberal and better suited to treating the conditions for detention, the conditions in the former were still "a lawful detention for a mentally unsound person" (§ 47), assessing the fact that the authorities had tried to find a solution, but were unable to do so (§ 48).

Reviewing the situation of the detention at reasonable intervals is required, as doing otherwise is a violation of Article 5.4 of the European Convention of Human Rights (*Silva Rocha v. Portugal*, § 32).

In any case, the law of precedent of the European Court of Human Rights is still surprising, by affirming the use of coercive methods such as forced-feeding, relative isolation (the patient was still able to have visitors and take walks), or even the use of handcuffs, which is concerning, as acknowledged by the Court, as not forming a basis of violation of Article 3 of the European Convention of Human Rights, since "in general, a measure pronounced as being medically necessary cannot be declared as being inhumane or degrading" (*Herczegfalvy v. Austria*, § 82).

Regarding the respect of privacy, a violation of Article 8 of the European Convention of Human Rights was recognized in *Herczegfalvy v. Austria* when a legally undisclosed interference had the hospital forward all of the patient's letters to his curator to decide whether or not these should be sent (§ 91).

3.4.4   The European Convention for the Prevention of Torture and Inhuman or Degrading Treatment or Punishment

The development of Article 3 of the European Convention of Human Rights was approved in Strasbourg by the Committee of Ministers, as the Convention for the Protection of Human Rights and Fundamental Freedoms on November 26, 1987, by which the European Committee for the Prevention of Torture and Inhuman or Degrading Treatment or Punishment (CPT) was created. The members of CPT are experts with outstanding ability and experience who must carry out their specific title's tasks independently and impartially.

This Committee, by means of periodical or additional visits if necessary, examines the treatment given to persons deprived of their liberty. Visits are carried out by two or more members in places of detention, such as prisons, juvenile detention centers, holding centers for immigration detainees, police stations, and psychiatric establishments. During the visits, the delegations have unlimited access to the places of detention, and are able to interview persons deprived of their liberty or anyone else they consider beneficial to provide information. After the visits, they formulate recommendations based on their observations, which are included in a report that is sent to the State concerned. This report constitutes a starting point for an ongoing dialogue with the State concerned.

The CPT also elaborates general reports on the subject matter that are encompassed in the "the CPT Standards." These documents are especially valuable with respect to involuntary psychiatric internments, civilly or criminally, and the Eighth General Report dealt specifically with this subject (CPT/Inf 98). Among the most notable aspects of the quoted Standards, the following questions stand out:

- **Staff**: Healthcare workers must be sufficient, experienced, and trained; auxiliary staff must be carefully chosen; caution must be taken when using patients as auxiliary staff.
- **Classification**: Necessary separation of adolescent patients from adult patients.

- **Living conditions**: Guarantee of basic needs, food, individualization of clothing and appropriate medication and environment, hygiene, lighting, heating and ventilation; space for each patient, a place to keep personal belongings, privacy in the bathrooms, closure of large-capacity dormitories, and access to their space during the day.
- **Treatment**: Based on an individualized integral plan, with a wide range of rehabilitative and therapeutic activities; supervision of prescription, and administration of psychiatric drugs; periodic reviews of the health condition and medications; electroconvulsive therapy must fit into the patient's treatment plan, and must be accompanied by appropriate safeguards, anesthetic and muscle relaxants, administered out of the view of other patients, by staff who have been specifically trained and who will document the treatments.
- **Documentation**: A personal medical file opened for each patient, allowing the patient access to it, unless it is therapeutically unadvisable.
- **Consent**: Consent must be the general rule, except in cases of clearly and strictly defined exceptional circumstances, based on the law. Internment is distinguished from treatment.
- **Information**: Complete, exact, and understandable on the patient's health condition and proposed treatment, informing the patient during the administration of such.
- **Coercive methods/measures**: Clearly defined policy for use with agitated or violent patients; giving preference to verbal instructions and only with the ineffectiveness of such would it be permissible to make use of physical restraints, basically manual control; the application is only by exception, as ordered by a doctor, not to be prolonged, and must be documented. Isolation should be at a minimum, guaranteeing adequate, and periodic human contact.
- **Involuntary internment**: The initial decision of placement must be made by a judicial authority, or at least guaranteeing an appeal before a judicial body. The patient must be informed of their rights and of the institution's internal routine, allowed to make complaints and communicate with others, especially with their lawyer. An independent outside body should make periodic visits, with the ability to speak privately with the patients, receive their complaints, and make recommendations that they regard as pertinent.
- **Discharge**: Discharge should be done as soon as the placement ceases to be necessary; the placement should not persist due to lack of adequate external facilities.

3.4.5 The Commissioner for Human Rights

This institution, created in 1999, serves as a complementary function to other human rights protection mechanisms. It is of a preventative nature and without jurisdictional authority.

The Commissioner for Human Rights elaborates annual reports for the countries on the state of the protection of human rights in Europe. It is worth mentioning the report elaborated by the Commissioner relating to the conditions of psychiatric internment in Romania, as it illustrates this institution's performance.

3.4.6   The European Convention on Human Rights and Biomedicine

The Convention for the protection of human rights and dignity with respect to Biology and Medicinal applications (Convention on Human Rights and Biomedicine) [15] was signed at Oviedo on April 4, 1997. It is one of the Council of Europe's most valuable instruments, as it links all the States that have ratified it.

It contains the following mandates, among others:

- Intervention of a person not able to consent must only take place when it is advantageous to their direct interest (Art. 6.1).
- In case of mental dysfunction which entails incompetence, the intervention may only be carried out with authorization from the representative, authorities, or a person or institution indicated by the law; the affected person should take part, as far as possible, in the authorization proceedings (Art. 6.3).
- Treatment of mental disorders without prior consent may only be carried out when there is a serious risk to the patient's health, and when respecting supervisory, control, and appeal procedures (Art. 7).
- In emergency situations, when prior consent cannot be obtained, necessary medical intervention may be carried out for the benefit of the affected person (Art. 8).
- The right for previously expressed wishes to be recognized (Art. 9).
- Restrictions on the exercise of rights to information about their own health, although only when in the interests of the patient, are allowed (Art. 10.3).
- Participation in scientific research of patients without the capacity to consent provided the following conditions are met: there is no alternative method, the risks are not disproportionate, the experiment must have been approved by a competent authority, the person is informed of their rights and guarantees, the anticipated results suppose a real personal and direct benefit to their health, the experiment cannot be carried out with comparable effectiveness on subjects capable of granting consent, and there is no objection by the concerned person (Art. 17.1). In the absence of a direct benefit, participation in research is only permitted if they meet the scrupulous conditions of Article 17.2.
- The extraction or removal of tissues and organs from persons without the capacity to consent is not permitted, except in exceptional cases, and adhering to rigorous conditions (Art. 20).

3.5   Other Organizations of Interest

3.5.1   The European Union

In the area of mental health care, the efforts of the EU fall short of those of the Council of Europe. There are some resolutions on the subject: European Parliament Resolution of December 14, 1995 on the human rights of disabled people (B4-1494, 1498, 1510, 1513, 1540 and 1552/95); European Parliament Resolution of May 23, 1996, on threats to the right to life of disabled persons (B4-0650/1996); Council Resolution of November 18, 1999 on the promotion of mental health (Official Journal C 86 of 24.03.2000); and Council Resolution of July15, 2003 on promoting the employment and social integration of people with disabilities (2003/C 175/01). Also cited are the Council Conclusions of June 2, 2003 on combating stigma and discrimination in relation to mental illness (Official Journal C 141, 17/06/2003 P.0001-0002); and the European Commission's Green Paper "Improving the mental health of the population: Towards a strategy on mental health for the European Union", of October 14, 1995.

The positive regulations are scarce as well as being very general. The consolidated version of the Constitutive Treaty of December 24, 2002, only dedicates Article 152 to public health, without any reference to the topic of mental health. The EU's Charter of Fundamental Rights, approved in Nice on July 7, 2000 is particularly applicable to the mentally ill population; Article 21.1, which proclaims the principle of non-discrimination, expressly mentions disability. Article 26 relates to the integration of persons with disabilities. Also worthy of mention is Article 3.2 which calls for particular respect to be paid in the field of medicine and biology to: "the free and informed consent of the person concerned, according to the procedures laid down by law." This most likely refers to "national" law.

The European Social Charter deserves a separate mention. This was signed in Turin on October 18, 1961 and entered into force on February 26, 1965. It contains several precepts related to mental health. Article 11 is devoted to the right to protection of health, committing the contracting States to eliminating the causes of ill health, to providing educational and consultative services for the promotion of health, to encouraging individual responsibility in matters of health, and to preventing epidemic, endemic, and other diseases as much as possible. Article 13 alludes to the right of social and medical assistance, guaranteeing that the people who do not dispose of sufficient resources may obtain adequate assistance. Finally, Article 15 refers to the right of physically or mentally handicapped persons to vocational training, and social and professional rehabilitation [16].

3.5.2   The World Health Organization Regional Office for Europe

The European Office of the WHO, approved a Declaration on the Promotion of Patients' Rights in Europe at a consultation held in Amsterdam on March 28–30, 1994. Considered therein are universally acknowledged patients' rights (informed consent prior to treatment, right to welfare information and to privacy). Noteworthy are the following: the presumption of consent in the case that the patient is incapable of expressing their wishes when it coincides with an emergency situation (3.3); the need to involve the patient, whether adult or minor, in the decision-making process as much as possible, including when the intervention of a representative is required (3.5); and a restriction on the intervention of incapacitated patients in clinical studies which do not offer them a direct benefit (3.10).

With regard to the supply of resources, the European Office organized a Ministerial Conference on "Mental Health: Facing Challenges, Building Solutions," in Helsinki from January 12–15, 2005. This drew the European States' attention to the need to allocate sufficient quality resources for mental health care.

3.5.3 European Studies on Better Legal Protection for Mental Patients

Recent studies have broached some of the most relevant questions regarding the protection of mental patients' rights, such as the "Placement and Treatment of Mentally Ill Offenders—Legislation and Practice in EU-Member States," promoted by the European Commission through its Directorate General for Health and Consumer Protection (DG SANCO), and the EUNOMIA Project (European Evaluation of Coercion in Psychiatry and Harmonization of Best Clinical Practice) sponsored by the European Union. These are proof of a renewed interest in this topic.

Resulting from some of the above, there are already publications in existence in the specific area of ethical-legal frameworks [7–9].

In the near future, new regulatory documents that improve on the measures for protection of mental patients have not been ruled out, either by way of agreement in the forum of the Council of Europe resulting in further recommendations, or through EU directives. In any case, it can be affirmed that the debate over the rights of mental patients in Europe is in progress and benefits from a high level of social and institutional involvement. Although it must be recognized that despite such important postulates, principles, and recommendations, there continues to be a significant deficit in implementation: a declarative plan does not always translate into practice.

3.5.4 Ethical Issues in European Forensic Psychiatry

Some European forensic psychiatrists are convinced that an element that differs between Europe and the United States with respect to ethics in forensic psychiatry is the idea that the forensic doctor's task is the care of the patient's well-being and that the experience and knowledge of a psychiatrist is medicinal, and as such forensic psychiatrists must respect the ethical principles of general medicine [5].

This idea is not shared by some American forensic psychiatrists as evidenced by the long debate stirred by the Stone-Appelbaum controversy [17–18]. They believe that there are two ways to focus forensic psychiatry with respect to ethical issues: one is to define forensic medicine as independent from general medicine because it lacks a true clinical medical relationship with the patient; and the other way is to regard it as sharing the same ethical codes approved by the Ethics Committee of the American Psychiatric Association, which declare that: "psychiatrists are physicians, and physicians are physicians at all times" (Ethical Principles of Psychologist and Code of Conduct. American Psychological Association, 1992) [19].

Thus it can be said that the problems encountered in mental health care in Europe, especially in the field of forensic psychiatry, do not differ greatly from those experienced in North America. Both face difficulties due to the variety of legislations (there are over 50 separate legal systems in the United States) [20].This means that dialogue and the exchange of experiences between the United States and the EU may be mutually very beneficial in developing new tools to improve mental health practices.

When talking about the differences, we must also refer to methodological questions. In Europe there is a propensity to assign a purely legal quality to ethical matters. The tendency is to look for solutions to ethical problems by resorting to the law, also evidenced by a culture that values human rights above all.

The topics of mental health and human rights receive a lot of attention from the media and European civilian society. There is a need for appropriate treatment on one side, and social rehabilitation on the other, so that the detainee afflicted with a mental illness may benefit from mental health services and the judicial system at the same time.

This aspect puts pressure on forensic research to find a way to satisfy both the need to preserve rights and to promote strategies that respond to the demand to offer adequate treatment. Despite this, in some States basic human rights may be restricted for security reasons. In The Netherlands, civil rights may be suspended in the case of detainees with mental disorders as with ordinary patients. Only in Austria, those detained with mental illnesses sentenced to more than a year in prison lose their right to vote if their sentencing evidences a criminal responsibility not attributed to their illness [10].

Regarding the debate over ethical issues, the North American cultural influence in Europe runs deep and is far-reaching. The *Declaration on the Promotion of Patient Rights in Europe* issued by the WHO European Regional Office has influenced all the subsequent guidelines issued by the Council of Europe. The ethical issues dealt with in the Declaration pertain to the cultural heritage of North American bioethics, which has greatly influenced European culture. Issues such as medical-patient relationships, informed consent, the right to refuse treatment, the right to a second opinion, the right to a written diagnosis on discharge, and the right to privacy [21] all form part of the common heritage between Europe and the United States.

In spite of the efforts made over the past few decades, differences among mental health systems remain as a great obstacle to the unification process. The importance of having a legal tool that fosters the development of reform is undeniable, but it is not in itself sufficient to bring about action in such a heterogeneous context.

The language of right, or law, possesses an intrinsic flexibility that permits an interpretation of norms according to different points of view. Its role is that of helping to reach an agreement among the parties offering minimum guarantees, such as equity and justice.

If the harmonization of the mental health system is accomplished solely through the creation of legal tools, the risk is that it will succeed in reducing the fragmentation in myriad national frameworks, and may allow Member States to interpret the laws according to the interests of those lobbying and the political groups in power. If mental health is governed exclusively by legislation, it might become a kind of defensive medicine, a consequence of the insecurity experienced by its providers because the criteria followed in practice are unclear. In such situations, the tendency is to find comfort and security in norms, forgetting that in the law, certainty is only achieved in the supreme tribunal, but in its absence, all norms are subject to interpretation. For this reason, a true harmonization of mental health systems cannot avoid generating new attitudes toward mental health seeking not only the realization of what is just, but also the pursuit of what is optimal.

References

1. Shorter, E. (2007) The historical development of mental health services in Europe, in *Mental Health Policy and Practice Across Europe: The Future Direction of Mental Health Care* (eds. M. Knapp, D. McDaid, E. Mossialos, and G. Thornicroft), Open University Press, McGraw-Hill, New York, pp. 15–33.
2. Thornicroft, G. and Tansella, M. (2004) Components of a modern mental health service: pragmatic balance of community and hospital care-overview of systematic evidence. *The British Journal of Psychiatry*, **185**, 283–90.
3. Marusic, A. (2004) Mental health in the enlarged European Union: need for relevant public mental action. *The British Journal of Psychiatry*, **184**, 450–1.
4. Becker, T. and Vázquez-Baquero, J.L. (2001) The European perspective of psychiatric reform. *Acta Psychiatrica Scandinavica*, **104** (410), 8–14.
5. Gordon, H. and Lindqvist, P. (2007) Forensic psychiatry in Europe. *Psychiatry Bulletin*, **31**, 421–4.
6. Fioritti, A. and Xavier, M. (2005) Background factors and underlying influences, in *Placement and Treatment of Mentally Disordered Offenders. Legislation and Practice in the European Union* (eds. H.J. Salize and H. Dressing), Pabst Scientific Publishers, Lengerich, pp. 29–33.
7. Dressing, H., Salize, H.J., and Gordon, H. (2007) Legal frameworks and key concepts regulating diversion and treatment of mentally disordered offenders in European Union member states. *European Psychiatry*, **22**, 427–32.
8. Dressing, H. and Salize, H.J. (2005) Forensic psychiatry, in *Placement and Treatment of Mentally Disordered Offenders. Legislation and Practice in the European Union* (eds. H.J. Salize and H. Dressing), Pabst Scientific Publishers, Lengerich, pp. 14–27.
9. Dressing, H. and Salize, H.J. (2006) Forensic psychiatric assessment in European Union members states. *Acta Psychiatrica Scandinavica*, **114**, 282–9.
10. Dressing, H., Salize, H.J., Ferrari, H., and Leue, A. (2005) Forensic psychiatry assessment, in *Placement and Treatment of Mentally Disordered Offenders. Legislation and Practice in the European Union* (eds. H.J. Salize and H. Dressing), Pabst Scientific Publishers, Lengerich, pp. 72–81.
11. Tuke, S. (1996) *Description of The Retreat, an institution near York, for insane persons of the Society of Friends. Containing an account of its origin and progress, the modes of treatment, and a statement of cases. With an elevation and plans of the building*, Process Press, London.
12. Álvarez, R., Huertas, R., and Peset, J.L. (1993) Enfermedad mental y sociedad en la Europa de la segunda mitad del siglo XIX. *Asclepio*, **45** (2), 41–60.
13. Colombier, J. and Doublet, F. (1785) Instructions sur la manière de gouverner les insensés et de travailler à leur guérison dans les asiles qui leur sont destinés, L'Imprimerie Royale, Paris (éd. original).
14. Pinel, P. (1801) *Traité médico-philosophique sur l'aliénation mentale ou la manie*, Richard, Caille & Ravier, Paris. 2nd edition, J.A. Brosson, Paris, 1809. [*A Treatise on Insanity* (transl. D.D. Davis). New York, Hafner, 1962.]
15. Salado, A. (1994) Las funciones del Comité europeo para la prevención de la tortura. *Revista de Instituciones Europeas*, **21** (2), 563–84.

16. De Burca G. and De White B. (eds.) (2005) *Social Rights in Europe*, Oxford University Press, New York/Oxford.

17. Stone, A.A. (1984) The ethical boundaries of forensic psychiatry: a view from the Ivory Tower. *Bulletin of the American Academy of Psychiatry and the Law*, **12**, 209–19.

18. Appelbaum, P.S. (1997) A theory of ethics for forensic psychiatry. *Bulletin of the American Academy of Psychiatry and the Law*, **25**, 233–47.

19. Nedopil, N. (2004) The boundaries of courtroom expertise. *Ethical issues in forensic psychiatry. Directions in Psychiatry*, **24**, 107–20.

20. Halpern, A.L. (2008) Can we harmonise forensic psychiatry across Europe? *The Psychiatrist*, **32**, 74.

21. Neelman, J. and Van Os, J. (1996) Ethical issues in European psychiatry. *European Psychiatry*, **11** (1), 1–6.

Part Two

The Practice of Forensic Psychiatry

4 The Forensic Psychiatric Examination

Robert L. Sadoff

University of Pennsylvania School of Medicine, Philadelphia, USA

4.1 Introduction

A number of books and articles have been written about how to conduct the forensic psychiatric examination [1–4]. This chapter will not duplicate those fine efforts. The purpose of this chapter is to introduce the concept of minimizing harm while conducting the forensic psychiatric examination. There are a number of areas in which the examination may prove to be harmful to the examinee (and sometimes to the examiner). There are vulnerable individuals and populations that are examined in a forensic context, for example, children, adolescents, elderly, mentally retarded, severely mentally ill, immigrants, victims of sexual abuse, or victims of workplace violence.

One of the ways of minimizing harm in conducting the examination is to recognize the vulnerability of the individual being examined and plan in advance to ease the anxiety, or minimize the tension the person will experience. This relates to the Appelbaum [5] concept of respect for the individual. In addition to giving the usual information to the examinee about who the examiner is and what will be done with the information obtained, the examiner should also make every effort to put the examinee at ease. If, for example, the examinee is a child under the age of 12 or 13, it is my preference to have a trained child forensic psychiatrist conduct the examination rather than one without training in child or adolescent psychiatry. If the examinee is a woman who has suffered from sexual abuse or aggravated rape, it behooves the examiner to approach the examination with sensitivity and respect. Sometimes, such a survivor of violent criminal behavior would want to be examined only by another female, or would want to have another person in the room with her during the examination. I often recommend female forensic

Ethical Issues in Forensic Psychiatry: Minimizing Harm   by Robert L. Sadoff
© 2011 John Wiley & Sons, Ltd

psychiatrists in such matters, and I have no problem in having a "chaperone" present to protect the interests of the examinee during the forensic assessment.

Simon and Wettstein [1] present the following 11 guidelines for conducting a forensic psychiatric examination:

1. maintain examiner objectivity and neutrality.
2. respect examinee autonomy.
3. protect confidentiality.
4. obtain informed consent.
5. interact verbally.
6. insure no previous, current, or future personal relations with the examinee.
7. avoid sexual contact.
8. preserve relative anonymity.
9. establish a clear fee policy.
10. provide a suitable examination setting.
11. define time and length of examination.

These are all important guidelines that are consistent with the sources of ethical principles in psychiatry and forensic psychiatry.

4.2 Exemplary Case

The idea for writing this book originated in a seminar that I lead at the University of Pennsylvania School of Medicine on "Practical Issues in Forensic Psychiatry." One of the child forensic psychologists gave a wonderful presentation of the examination of a young girl caught in a domestic relations controversy. She had accused her father of sexually abusing her and had to be examined by a number of people as part of the divorce proceedings and the child custody assessment ordered by the court. The child had been examined on several prior occasions and had shown negative reactions to such examinations, becoming hysterical, crying, and running from the room.

When the child forensic psychologist presented the information to our seminar, she asked herself how she could conduct this examination with a minimal amount of trauma to the youngster while obtaining sufficient information in order to complete her assignment as ordered by the court. She considered a number of different options in preparation for a very difficult examination of an extremely vulnerable individual. It was her sensitivity and experience in working with children that allowed her to reach a compromise where she would minimize the trauma to the child while obtaining sufficient data to present to the court. She allowed the mother to be present during the first two examinations in order to become comfortable with the examiner, and then saw the child alone, so there would be no accusation of inappropriate influence by the mother on the child's responses.

The examiner had some concern about the accuracy or veracity of the accusations against the father and wanted to observe the child in the company of her father, but knew that could be a traumatizing experience for the child. She prepared for the confrontation in her office by spending time with the child, discussing the father with the child, and preparing the child for the combined examination of the child and her father. To her surprise, she found the child was quite taken with the father, and the experience proved to be therapeutic rather than traumatic for the child.

I was tremendously impressed with the professionalism of the psychologist who conducted this very difficult assessment by utilizing her skills and her experience in preparing the child and minimizing any trauma that could have occurred without such sensitivity and respect for the youngster. I believe that we could learn from this experience and generalize to other examinations in order to minimize the inherent harm in the work we do.

4.3 Third Parties in the Examination

There are a number of colleagues who resist having a third party present during an examination, insisting that it "dilutes the purity of the examination." Many of these people will teach and have students present during their demonstration examinations and do not consider that to be a "dilution of purity." However, it is my opinion that they are threatened by the presence of an attorney or another person in the room who would take notes during the examination and perhaps critique the exam at some later point, especially in court under cross-examination. The forensic examiner should have no concern about such a procedure or process. It is part of the adversarial system, and if the examiner respects the examinee and minimizes the harm through sensitive questioning, there should be no repercussions within the adversary process.

There are times, however, when an aggressive attorney, sitting with his or her client, becomes intrusive and obstructionistic, interfering with the smooth process of conducting the examination. In those cases, the attorney should be instructed that he or she is not allowed to interfere with the examination, but, clearly, if the attorney feels the question is harmful to their client, he or she has every right to object, and perhaps ask the examiner to word the question in a different manner.

Simon [6] is concerned about third parties being present in the examination and believes that the forensic psychiatric examination is conducted best in privacy. He points out that forensic psychiatrists must consider the skewing effects of having third parties present during the independent psychiatric examination. He quotes Zonana: "The psychiatric interview is not merely a set of questions and answers; it is a complex integration of many sources of data that include verbal response, style, reaction, and quality of interaction. Any factors which alter the way in which a psychiatrist collects and experiences the data alter the validity of the interpretation of the data in one way" [7].

Simon also notes, "The presence of the attorney representing the examinee may impart an added adversarial tone and chill the examination, making it difficult for the forensic psychiatrist to develop an examination rapport with the examinee ... The presence of attorneys may also provide an occasion for the examinee to magnify symptoms, either consciously or unconsciously" [6]. Simon also notes that the presence of the examinee's family members or friends may provide added psychological support.

My own experience involves the examination of well over 10 000 individuals, and I have held several hundred with attorneys present, especially when I was conducting either an independent medical examination, in civil cases, for the defense, or an examination, in criminal cases, for the prosecution. On only one occasion did I have to ask the attorney to leave, because he was so intrusive and interfered excessively with the examination. Mostly, attorneys are quite respectful, and if the examiner shows similar respect to the client, there is no need for interference or obstructionism. Abusive attorneys could well be reported to the judge involved in the case, and would then have to defend their intrusive actions during the examination, and perhaps be reprimanded if the judge felt their actions were inappropriate and excessive.

4.4 Seeking Truth and Justice

It is important for the forensic examiner to recognize his or her role in conducting these examinations. Ideally, forensic experts should have no interest in the outcome of the case and, therefore, should not have any "axe to grind" one way or the other when it comes to conducting the examination. They do the best job they are able to do under the circumstances, protecting their integrity and their professionalism, but not becoming involved as an adversary, as too many of our colleagues have done in the past. It is not our job to argue the case or to reach a conclusion that our retaining attorney would like, but rather to provide professional medical psychological information that is not available to the average intelligent lay person, and that we have the experience and expertise to provide in the interests of justice. That is the second arm of our ethical duty, which is to seek truth and justice and to strive for objectivity and neutrality rather than bias or favoritism.

Here we have a juxtaposition of the two ethical duties of the forensic examiner: respect for the individual and seeking truth or justice. In the case of a victim of sexual abuse, criminal rape, or other serious sensitive violent crime, how much detail does the examiner require from the victim, who is now the examinee, in order to reach a meaningful conclusion? Do examiners need to have victims relate, in excruciating detail, the experience that they have had that led to the lawsuit or to the criminal charges against the defendant? Is there a deposition transcript the examiner can review in conducting a complete assessment of the person? If so, attorneys notoriously ask very detailed questions on cross-examination for a number of reasons, mostly to get the details that are important for their case. Sometimes, attorneys will push to have the victim relate embarrassing and sensitive details, because they are painful and the attorney is not sensitive to the pain of the victim who is on "the other side" of the adversarial system. If one has such a transcript, then in my opinion examiners do not need to put victims through the ordeal of every excruciating detail that will again be painful, and have examinees "relive" the horrifying experiences that were so traumatic for them.

Of course, examiners can be criticized on cross-examination for not getting all the details when they reached their opinion. Suppose, for example, the examiner is sensitive to the needs of the victim and does not insist on having him or her relate every detail and reaches the conclusion for the defense, in a civil case, that the victim was traumatized, but the trauma did not lead to a post-traumatic stress disorder (PTSD), as the plaintiff's expert had concluded. On cross-examination, the plaintiff's attorney may accuse the defense expert of "cutting corners" by not getting all the details. In essence, the attorney would be punishing the expert for being sensitive and kind to their client by not putting him or her through the ordeal of relating all the details of their trauma. Nevertheless, the defense expert could explain to the court that it was not felt necessary to re-traumatize the plaintiff by putting him or her through that ordeal and would appear to be a sensitive, helpful medical professional rather than an adversary. Since the defense expert's opinion does not help the plaintiff's case, the expert would be seen as more neutral rather than advocating for the defense position.

However, we then come to an area that has been critiqued by Stone [8] about the "seductiveness" of the examiner, who is seen by the plaintiff as being a medical person and, therefore, helpful. Plaintiffs may give information to such a helpful medical individual that hurts their case and supports the conclusion and opinion of the defense expert. In the environment of a helpful and therapeutic interview, plaintiffs may downgrade the impact of the trauma on their psychological symptoms, thereby supporting the conclusion of the examiner that they had a terrible trauma, but were able to react to it without serious emotional consequences.

On balance, I would opt for the humanitarian approach of the sensitive (though possibly "seductive") examiner rather than the one who is obsessive and compulsively meticulous about getting every detail of the trauma, even though it is painful and harmful to the examinee. Is there a middle ground? Can examiners obtain sufficient information without overly traumatizing victims and without becoming seductive and misleading plaintiffs in their recitation of their symptoms and how they relate to the trauma experienced? I would hope that each of us conducting such examinations with vulnerable individuals would seek that middle ground that would minimize the harm to our examinee (showing respect, according to the Appelbaum [5] doctrine) while obtaining sufficient information in order to seek truth and justice (also the Appelbaum ethical approach). Thus, in such cases, we may not be able to "first, do no harm," but we certainly can minimize the harm that is inherent in the work we do in order to complete our assignment.

4.5   Malingering

There are some psychiatrists who work exclusively for the defense in civil cases, who insist on having all the details, primarily because they are concerned about malingering and want to look for consistency of details of the trauma from one reporting to the next. Initially, there is the official complaint that is filed and the statement the individual gives to the police or the authorities. There is then the deposition transcript that should be reviewed in civil cases, and when it exists, in criminal cases. Mostly, the attorneys questioning the defendant or plaintiff, will obtain meticulous details about the trauma or the criminal behavior. It may not be necessary in all cases for the examining psychiatrist to put the plaintiff through the trauma of reliving the horrible experiences again during the examination. On the other hand, the mental health professional retained by the defense may feel it necessary to get all the details in order to compare with what the plaintiff testified on deposition or at preliminary hearing in the case of a defendant in a criminal case.

4.6   Sensitivity v. Thoroughness

When conducting the forensic examination, one should be as thorough as possible even when not subjecting the plaintiff, or the defendant in a criminal case, to excruciating details that may be harmful in repeating over and over again. This is especially important when the examination is being recorded for the opposing psychiatrist to review.

In one particular case, the expert for the prosecution agreed with the two experts for the defense, one psychiatrist and one psychologist, that the defendant suffered from a significant mental disorder, and they all agreed that it was schizophrenia with an affective component or a diagnosis of schizoaffective disorder. The two defense experts concluded that the defendant acted on his command hallucinations, as part of his mental disorder, that commanded him to kill his girlfriend because the voices told him that she was plotting to kill him. The prosecution expert, agreeing that there was a serious mental disorder, did not agree with the conclusion about criminal responsibility. The prosecution expert stated, in his report, that the defendant did not link his mental illness with his criminal behavior and, therefore, was not legally insane. The expert said, in the report, if the defendant had indicated that the girlfriend had been plotting to kill him and, therefore, he had to kill her as he had told the defense experts, then the prosecution expert would have concluded that the defendant was criminally insane under the guidelines of that jurisdiction. However, the expert concluded there was no such linkage.

Upon reviewing the videotape and the transcript of the examination by the prosecution expert, it was noted that as the defendant was explaining how this group of people was plotting to kill him, he was interrupted by the examiner, asking questions that distracted him from his narration about what had occurred and why he killed his girlfriend. They never did return to the subject, and the defendant was not able to tell the prosecution examiner what he had told the other two defense experts that included the girlfriend in the plot to kill him.

The examination was seen as incomplete. It was also seen as biased inasmuch as the prosecution expert would have concluded, as the other two experts had, that the defendant was insane and he would have received treatment for his mental illness rather than punishment for the "murder" that the prosecution expert delineated in his report. It was also seen as a reflection of his bias to utilize the term "murder" rather than homicide. It could be manslaughter, or it could be killing without criminal responsibility, as in insanity.

This example is utilized to illustrate how harm can come when the examination is incomplete or when the examiner's bias intrudes on the effectiveness of the examination, leading to a distorted conclusion. It is also a reflection of how important it is to videotape or record examinations conducted by adversarial experts.

4.7   Dangers of Being Too Sensitive to the Examinee

In a civil case, one of the dangers of not asking all the specific questions that may harm the plaintiff further is to miss the important details that might be significant in evaluating mental illness, malingering, or manipulation of the data. One may be criticized for failing to ask pertinent questions in order to save the examinee from excessive anxiety.

Another danger in being overly sensitive is that the very nice, sensitive professional approaching the defendant in a criminal case, or the plaintiff in a civil case, may be overly seductive in his or her approach and allow the examinee to drop their guard and give more information than they had intended or were willing to give. There have been many occasions where I have obtained information from plaintiffs in civil cases, or defendants, in criminal cases, when working for "the other side" that was not obtained by the expert for their side. For some reason, they found it necessary or comfortable to open up and give information that they had once either withheld or were never asked.

One of the important issues is whether questions are asked. Plaintiffs and defendants are instructed by their attorneys to answer only the questions that are asked and not to provide excessive or extra information to the examiner. That is a wise instruction that should always be followed by all clients. However, there are some individuals who like to talk, and will do so if they feel they have a "friendly ear." That is why it is so important for examining professionals to provide the examinee with the information about who they are, their role in the adversarial process, and the consequences that may occur to the examinee.

One example of this type of information given to "the other side" occurred in a federal criminal case. I had examined a woman for the defense and found that she was seriously mentally ill and met the federal standard for the insanity defense. She was examined by a very skilled forensic psychiatrist for the prosecution who obtained even more data and more information than I was able to get, and he concluded that she was seriously mentally ill and also reached the opinion that she met the standard for the insanity defense. His recommendation for treatment was specific and detailed. This may be considered a therapeutic forensic examination by the opposing expert.

In another similar case, I had examined for the defense a woman who had killed one of her parents in a psychotic frenzy. I concluded that she was mentally ill and also met the standard for the insanity defense in that jurisdiction. The state appointed a very skilled and experienced forensic psychiatrist to examine this woman and allowed me to be present during his examination. I was quite impressed with his thoroughness and the information he was able to obtain from her, reaching a conclusion that she was even more seriously psychotic than I had believed, and gave an opinion about her need for treatment and also that she had met the standard for insanity in that state. What is important here is the ability to obtain information, even when working "for the other side," if one approaches the examinee in a professional manner, with respect, and minimizes the harm through sensitive questioning.

4.8   Exaggeration or Malingering

Forensic psychiatrists and psychologists are often called on to provide opinions and render testimony in which minor head trauma, accompanied by persistent somatic, cognitive, and/or emotional symptoms, is alleged. The frequency of persistent symptoms following such minor head injury is generally low. The forensic clinician therefore must differentiate between subtle brain dysfunction, symptom amplification or psychogenic bases as the cause for the presence of cognitive and other deficits, or frank malingering. How does one differentiate between the exaggeration or the bona fide symptoms following head injuries? One must have a healthy degree of skepticism, though not cynicism. The use of psychological testing may help in terms of the subtle neuropsychological changes that may not be detected on gross neurological testing, such as the CAT scan, MRI, or PET scan. The point here is not to harm the plaintiff by disbelieving him or her just because one is working for the defense. The examiner must do a complete and thorough job. Consistency of symptoms and credibility of symptoms related to the degree of head trauma must be considered.

4.8.1   Case Example

In one case, the examiner gave an opinion that the driver of the motor vehicle could not have sustained such a serious blow to the head since the damage to the automobile was minor. That is not a scientific way of assessing brain damage. In that particular case, the plaintiff was clearly injured and did sustain not only cognitive impairment, but emotional disturbance, both of which required treatment. To indicate that the plaintiff was not injured in the motor vehicle accident and, therefore, does not have a bona fide claim to psychological damage, would be harmful to the plaintiff and may deprive him or her of necessary treatment. Similarly, evaluating an individual who has been in treatment following such a brain injury will often require regular assessments to determine the effect of treatment and whether there is improvement, and to what degree. Examining individuals in therapy and determining that they never sustained a bona fide injury and are not in need of such treatment can also be harmful if, in fact, there is need for treatment, because the damage was sustained and the person has shown improvement with treatment. Stopping the treatment prematurely, because there is improvement, can also be harmful to the claimant.

In a similar manner, an assessor may fail to diagnose PTSD if the examiner underestimates the plaintiff's pathology or assumes the plaintiff has "a normal reaction" to the event in question. Inadequate time spent with the plaintiff may also result in missing the correct diagnosis. Another source of error might be the confusion caused by a preexisting condition with a recent onset of PTSD. Sometimes, people who have preexisting conditions are more vulnerable to a follow-up traumatic event that causes serious emotional damage, including symptoms of PTSD. Just because a person had a prior injury that may have caused emotional symptoms, does not necessarily negate the effect of the current trauma on the individual.

4.9 Injury and Disability

There are four different levels of concern following an injury or an accident. First, there is the event in question, which may be a motor vehicle accident, an aggravated rape, or other serious physical event. The second level is that the accident or incident led to injury to the person involved. The third level is that the injury then led to impairment in function so that the plaintiff was not able to work as effectively as previously because of the emotional consequences of the event in question. Finally, there is the concept of disability, which is determined by a disability board assessing the degree of impairment and its relationship to the event.

The forensic expert has the responsibility of examining the plaintiff with respect to the damage that may have been caused by the event. The assessment of injury is determined by the symptoms presented that either are or are not consistent with the degree of physical injury or the emotional impact of the event in question. The forensic expert must then determine whether that injury has led to impairment of function. That is usually determined by the subjective evaluation of the plaintiff indicating to the examiner what impact the injury has had on their ability to function in various areas. Sometimes, as we have seen, the plaintiff will exaggerate symptoms, or lie about them, or malinger, and there are ways of determining when a person is malingering. Some will use videotape surveillance, and others will utilize lie detector tests, a battery of psychological tests, or the inconsistency of symptoms with the injury noted.

Therefore, it behooves the forensic examiner to have available the work record of the individual to determine what their performance was like before the injury and following the injury. Are the psychological tests consistent with the impairment claimed? The disability policy may be written for the specific professional function the individual has performed. For example, a neurosurgeon who injures a hand is unable to practice neurosurgery, but could do other work in the medical profession.

4.9.1 Case Example

A case example is that of a surgeon who was playing basketball and was elbowed in the eye going up for a rebound. The injury caused eye damage and visual difficulties. He noted problems with three-dimensional vision, and was not able to focus effectively or operate clearly. He was examined by an insurance doctor for the defense who gave him "a clean bill of health" and said that his visual acuity was not so bad that he could not operate. The surgeon then asked the evaluator whether the evaluator would want the surgeon to operate on the evaluator's mother if she had a particular problem in his specialty. The examiner confessed that he would not, and then changed his opinion about whether the surgeon had a disability.

Experts who see no damage to people, or believe that people generally are malingering or faking their illness, may harm plaintiffs who would then not be able to collect for disability even though they are not able to work. If professional examiners are going to call plaintiffs malingerers or a liars, they should at least have evidence, and not just label them because they work for the defense and usually do not find illness in those they examine. It has been my experience that there is pressure on the part of defense attorneys or insurance companies to find psychiatrists who will agree with their position in not finding illness or disability. I have had the experience of conducting a number of independent medical examinations and find that in many of the cases there is impairment, and I recommended treatment for the individual with the disability. After I gave such opinions, in a few cases, the referrals from that insurance company stopped coming in. Unfortunately, there are those who depend upon such referrals for their livelihood and on repeat evaluations from various insurance companies or defense attorneys. They may lose those referrals if they find too many cases of disability or impairment. I do not want to sound cynical, but I do point out the pressures that are on the forensic examiner, who is pledged to seek truth and justice and to act in an honest, unbiased manner.

There is a similar condition with prosecutors who want to find "neutral" forensic psychiatrists and not those who always find mental illness that would account for criminal behavior and, in some way, either excuse or justify it, if not just explain it. Clearly, there are many people who have serious mental illnesses who are still competent to proceed and are not legally insane for the criminal behavior. Unfortunately, I have found too many colleagues who tend to find in the direction their retaining attorney is headed.

When assessing a person with respect to disability and returning to work, forensic experts should be familiar with the job that has to be done to determine whether their examinee is capable of performing such work. Sometimes, I have conducted collateral interviews of people who work in the same position. I have also visited the place of work in order to view for myself the environment which the plaintiff has claimed to be "toxic." Specialists in workplace injuries and vocational rehabilitation experts may be consulted for definitive recommendations.

4.10   Harm to the Examiner

When discussing harm, we usually concern ourselves with the harm that can be caused to the examinee. I have also considered harm to the examiner, or the professional, either in conducting the examination, in writing the report, or in testifying in court. Another harm to consider is that to the profession itself when experts become "hired guns," giving opinions solely for the money to be obtained. Dattilio [9] and others have written on the attitudes of lawyers who prefer experts who give opinions primarily for one side or the other rather than those experts who are seen to be objective and striving for neutrality. In many cases, attorneys do select "neutral" psychiatrists, those who have worked for both sides and are considered to be credible and honest. However, there are a number of attorneys who prefer to predict what their experts are going to say before hiring them. Those with a track record of working primarily for the prosecution or the defense in criminal cases, or the plaintiff or defense in civil cases, are usually sought by the attorneys working in that direction.

4.10.1   Case Example—Civil Trauma

I recently encountered a man who lost his son and mother in a tragic auto accident. He mourned their loss and was extremely angry at the drunk driver who hit them in a head-on collision. He had difficulty in mourning the loss of his loved ones, but continued to work and take care of the rest of his family. He took no medication, sought no treatment until he was involved in another accident about a year after the death of his family members. After that accident, in which he was not physically injured, he developed severe depression and symptoms of PTSD. He then sought treatment, was placed on an antidepressant medication and continued his therapy. In his lawsuit against the driver of the other car, he claimed serious emotional damage. The defense attorney, believing that most of his depression was due to the loss of his mother and son, called a psychiatrist to evaluate him and his claim that his current depression was due exclusively or primarily to the auto accident that rekindled his previous feelings of loss after the deaths of his loved ones.

I was asked to conduct this examination for the defense, and knew that it would be a sensitive experience and that he would be upset and perhaps angry and mistrusting because I represented the defense, who was trying to show that he did not have damage from this accident. I reviewed all the records and prepared to see him. He was clearly quite upset and depressed and angry, and his attorney accompanied him to the examination, but did not interfere in any way. Initially, he was rather resistant, quite angry, and defensive. I had given him the usual statements, who I represented, what I was going to do with the information he gave me, and what effect that would have upon him. These are statements of limited confidentiality which are necessary in conducting a forensic examination.

When I did not challenge him and his assertions as the attorneys did at his deposition two weeks before, he softened, became less defensive, and more cooperative in the examination. Indeed, I found that his symptoms had recurred after the auto accident and without that accident, he had been on the road to recovery, working and caring for the remainder of his family. Whether he would have become depressed ultimately, even without his later accident, one cannot say within reasonable medical certainty. What I could, and did say in my report was that he was clearly affected by the loss of his loved ones, but he had begun to heal on his own until he had a similar traumatic experience that brought back all the old feelings and the old memories that he could not deal with on his own as he had before. He did require treatment, which was helpful to him, and it was my opinion that his recent accident was a significant factor in his current mental state.

Although that was not what the defense attorney wanted in the report, it was my opinion that that was accurate, it was valid, and it would be therapeutic for him, shortening the time of his treatment and, hopefully, helping him to accept the balance that occurs in these cases. It was not an all or none matter; I did not say, as his expert did, that all of his current feelings were related to his accident, but I did indicate that though it was difficult to parse out, there were significant events that one could look at in terms of his current mental state. These were his nightmares, his flashbacks to his recent accident, which always included the deaths of his mother and son, and his increased visits to the cemetery to see them. The treatment notes of his therapist, who was not his expert witness, clearly revealed the healing process had occurred following the deaths of his loved ones, but then his symptoms returned even more strongly after his own accident.

4.11   Therapeutic Examinations

Sometimes, we find, during the course of conducting forensic examinations, that the individual is quite seriously ill, acutely suicidal, and requires immediate treatment. On one occasion, a woman expressed her wish to kill herself because she could no longer tolerate the stress of awaiting trial on charges that she felt were inappropriate, exaggerated or false. She threatened to kill herself when she left my office. I was examining her for the prosecution, and she was quite open in her communications to me, but confessed that she did not tell her attorney or her own psychiatrist how seriously depressed and suicidal she was.

I felt an obligation to help this woman, even though my assignment was to examine her for the prosecution and to render an opinion about her state of mind with respect to competency to stand trial and criminal responsibility. I could not let her leave the office knowing that she was acutely suicidal and would likely kill herself if allowed. I called her attorney and told him that I felt he should come down and be with her when she left the office, because I was concerned about her welfare and her life. He did come down with a female associate attorney, and they took responsibility for her when she left my office, calming her down and ultimately taking her to a nearby emergency room for evaluation and assessment. She was seen to be suicidal and hospitalized. I did not see her disclosures to me as manipulative in order to obtain a better result with the court. I felt she was sincere in her wish to harm herself, and I could not allow that to happen. Thus, forensic psychiatric assessments may not only minimize harm, but may also prevent future disaster.

4.11.1   Case Examples

A dramatic experience occurred in the assessment of a young college student who was accused of killing a classmate. He had been seen by two very experienced and respected forensic psychiatrists, one for the defense and one for the prosecution, both of whom felt that there was no significant mental illness in the defendant. The family, in a desperate effort, called my office and asked if I would examine their son, who was confined in a local jail in another state. I agreed to go, and found the youngster seriously deteriorating , becoming psychotic, and I was concerned that he had a dissociative identity disorder (DID) that prevented him from recalling any details of the homicide for which he had been charged. I had access to all the notes and records of the two other psychiatrists and also spoke with the psychologist, in his hometown, who had treated him for anxiety when he was a high school student. I learned that he had dissociative events and memory losses, with loss of time that was not due to substance abuse. The one factor that did not fit with DID was that there was no history—at least apparently—of any early childhood sexual abuse.

Nevertheless, I wanted to return with an expert in the diagnosis of DID to be certain of the diagnosis before giving up on this youngster as the other two psychiatrists previously had done. When asking the prosecutor to return with the expert to conduct an extensive assessment, we were told that time was up, that we had all had our chance to conduct our assessment and evaluation, and we would not be permitted any further examinations. I suggested to the prosecutor that his role was to seek justice, and that we may have a very important consideration here that, if true, he would need to know about.

He reluctantly agreed to allow us to conduct this examination, but only on the conditions that he be present during the examination and that he could videotape our interviews and examination. The family refused to have the prosecutor (who was seen by them as the enemy) present at the examination, but I insisted that the prosecutor had never seen a person with DID in the past and if I were correct about the diagnosis, we would have a benefit in terms of a reasonable plea agreement. The family agreed, and it was clear that the diagnosis was DID. It was essential that the prosecutor was present and that it was all recorded on videotape from the outset. Five alters emerged, one of whom admitted to the killing and also discussed the sexual abuse that was clearly present, but hidden because of the psychotic delusions of the defendant.

Giving up on this youngster would have been harmful to him, but pushing a sensitive and agreeable prosecutor to be reasonable in seeking justice rather than winning a criminal case, proved to be helpful to the youngster, who was given a reasonable sentence on plea negotiation. The family was in agreement with the lower sentence (rather than life imprisonment without parole), and the youngster was sent to a facility within the state where his DID could be treated by staff who had experience in treating such conditions. The victim's family was also relieved that the case did not go to court, because information about their son, the victim, would have been embarrassing to the family if it had been allowed to be presented in open court. This case has been properly disguised and many specific details have been omitted in order to protect the privacy of the individuals involved. Clearly, this was a tragic case for all concerned. However, the important factor is the diminished harm to the defendant and his family as well as the victim's family.

The prosecutor, who was sensitive and cooperative, did obtain a conviction, but at the lesser degree that would allow for treatment and recovery of the defendant. It is sometimes important to be persuasive in pursuing justice. Follow-up reports indicate the defendant is improving with specific treatment in the correctional facility.

4.12 Therapeutic Forensic Examinations and Assessments

We have seen how forensic psychiatric examinations may be harmful to the examinee, or even to the professional examiner. However, such examinations can also be therapeutic or beneficial without officially being part of a therapy program. It is important for the forensic examiner to alert the examinee that the assessment is not for the purposes of therapy, but for legal purposes. However, there are times when it is necessary for the forensic psychiatrist or psychologist to act as a therapist while conducting a prolonged assessment over time in order to prevent harm to the plaintiff in a civil case, or the defendant in a criminal case.

4.12.1 Case Examples

An example of this type of emergency therapeutic assessment occurred when I examined a 30-year-old intelligent professional man who had been injured in a serious automobile accident during which he had been rendered paraplegic. He suffered a spinal injury that caused him to live his life in a wheelchair and be unable to walk. He also had bowel and bladder problems and became extremely depressed with suicidal rumination on a regular basis. He confided to me, as the forensic examiner, that he was seriously considering suicide after he won his civil case so that he would have sufficient money to give to his family before he died. He felt very angry at the drunk driver of the other car that had plowed into him at 70 miles per hour, causing him serious injuries. In addition, the passenger in his car was killed, and he felt responsible for her death. He had been working as a chemist in a laboratory, requiring him to do a lot of standing and walking. He was not able to continue his profession, and the passenger who was killed was his fiancée. He became morose, extremely depressed, and suicidal.

I felt compelled to consult with his attorney and confide in him about his suicidal potential, which I felt was real and that if he were successful in his lawsuit for him, that he would lose his client as he was contemplating suicide. I recognized this attorney as a sensitive and helpful individual who was there to help his clients. He agreed that we had to do something to keep him alive. He hired him as a legal assistant and put him through law school, hiring him as his associate following his graduation at the top of his class. He began therapy with another psychiatrist, thought about suicide, but began to feel more worthwhile, and he decreased the intensity of his suicidal urges. I continued to conduct a "prolonged evaluation" over several years in order to keep my report "up to date," but meanwhile offering therapeutic contact with him during this prolonged assessment phase. The trial was necessarily delayed in order for him to complete his studies, become an associate and abandon his suicidal wishes.

This is an example of the kind of creative therapeutic forensic assessment that can occur despite the fact that forensic evaluations are not necessarily part of therapy, but "a striving for justice."

On another occasion, a woman going through a divorce proceeding and feeling very frustrated, anxious, and depressed, left my office after the second evaluation session claiming she was going to crash her sports car into a tree and kill herself. I prevented her from leaving the office (because, presumably, I was bigger and stronger than she was and could physically restrain her, if necessary). I called her attorney, with whom she was very close, and he came over with a female associate with whom our client examinee had been working closely, and the three of them went out to dinner. She was calmed in her anxiety and tension by her attorneys, and no further outbursts occurred. I could have called the police or 911 to have her committed as a potential suicide, but I felt in her best interest, because it was an impulsive move that would not be sustained, the aid given by her attorneys was the proper, helpful action to take.

These are examples of how assessments, interviews, or examinations can be therapeutic, can also minimize harm or, in some cases, even eliminate harm.

Perlin [10] has written extensively about the civil rights of mental patients and is arguably the most prolific writer on mental health law. He has advocated that forensic psychiatrists and mental health professionals must adhere to the civil rights of the patient in conducting forensic examinations and not allow harm to come to the patient if possible. In a seminar that Professor Perlin gave at the University of Pennsylvania, he discussed a Russian man who had been confined at a forensic psychiatric hospital. The man did not speak English, and had been confined for several years, having been accused of killing his brother. He was thought to be catatonic, because he did not speak, and was considered to be incompetent to stand trial. It was Professor Perlin who had seen the letters "CCCP" on something the man had written, and Perlin recognized that it was Russian, so he called in a Russian Orthodox priest to communicate with him in his native language.

The priest was able to talk with the man, obtain information, and when Professor Perlin pursued the issue, he was able to find a 25-year-old newspaper account about the man who killed his brother because his brother had been having sex with the man's wife, and approached him with a knife. The defendant disarmed his brother and kept the brother from killing him, but in the process had stabbed his brother, leading to the brother's death. The concern here was one of self-defense. However, his stay in the forensic hospital was harmful to the man, because nobody bothered to obtain a proper translator, as nobody knew what his background was, since he was not talking. It was only because an attorney interested in civil rights of the mentally ill was able to break the code and find the proper information that the man did go to trial and was found not guilty based on self-defense.

A similar situation occurred when I was consulting at another forensic psychiatric hospital. A Russian patient was presented to me in the forensic psychiatric conference. Everyone at the hospital believed the man was incompetent, because they could not understand what he was talking about. He did not speak English, and no one at the hospital spoke Russian. I insisted on having a Russian interpreter aid in the examination and I determined the man was not mentally ill and that his being arrested and brought to the hospital was a "big mistake," because nobody understood him. In this case, the forensic examination was helpful within the hospital, because his civil rights had been violated due to a communication problem that was readily and easily resolved by use of a translator or interpreter.

4.13   Special Testing in Forensic Cases

With respect to doing special testing in forensic cases, I used to do sodium amytal interviews, which were considered "truth serum," primarily to help recover memory that a person claims to have lost at the time of the particular event, either an accident in a civil case or a violent episode in a criminal case. The use of sodium amytal is not without its side effects such as epiglottal spasm in 1% of the cases. I had done well over 150 cases using sodium amytal and had one episode of epiglottal spasm, which was treated effectively by the anesthesiologist, who was always present during the procedure.

I stopped doing the sodium amytal interviews when I found a hypnotherapist who was excellent and could induce hypnosis in most individuals he encountered. We did about 150 hypnotic interviews as well, and sometimes the results were harmful to the individual. In many cases of criminal behavior where defendants could not remember what happened at the time of the crime, they were able to remember under the effects of hypnosis, and the results often were not helpful to them. However, in many cases, the results were helpful.

One case involved a woman who had killed her husband, and the hypnosis was extremely helpful in that it showed she had regressed to the age of 10, where she had impotent rage toward her stepfather, who had sexually abused her on a repeated basis. It was during a period of such regression to the age of 10 that she equated her husband with her stepfather sexually abusing their son. She battered him, and had no memory of the event until hypnosis. She was acquitted on the basis of insanity and has recovered quite well with proper treatment.

4.14   Dangers to the Forensic Examiner

Another aspect of reducing harm is protecting the examiner during forensic psychiatric examinations. One example is that of an individual in another state who was thought to have a DID. I was asked to conduct the examination by a female forensic psychologist who contacted the retaining attorney asking to have me as part of the defense forensic team. The defendant had been accused of raping and killing several women over a period of many months, until he was apprehended. He was actually in jail on rape charges, for which he received 35 years in prison, during which time one of his alters confessed to the police that he was also the rape murderer they were seeking.

I insisted that if I were to conduct this examination in a prison that I was not familiar with, I would want some protections and precautions taken. I insisted that he be handcuffed, shackled at his ankles, and chained to the floor, because he was a man who stood 6′ 5″ and weighed about 300 pounds. I was no match for this man if he became violent. The host personality was a passive, bright, responsive, and compliant man of about 40 years of age. However, after about an hour into the interview and examination, I noticed an abrupt switch to an amoral, hostile, violent individual who lunged at the psychologist, threatening to rape her and to kill me. Fortunately, he was not able to reach us, because he was shackled and chained to the floor. Had we not taken these precautions, I may not be here to write this tale.

Examiners are at risk sometimes of being attacked or harmed during a forensic examination. Examiners should protect themselves from harm, but cannot always anticipate or foresee the danger. We have had a number of tragedies where psychiatrists have been killed by their patients.

I recall taking precautions in conducting one assessment of a man involved in a domestic relations dispute who told me, in the course of the assessment, that he carries a gun with him at all times. I told him I could not continue the examination while he had the gun in his pocket, because I would feel uncomfortable that he may attack me or kill me. He assured me that he would not do so, but I told him that he would have to leave his gun at home if I were to continue the assessment. He said he could not do that because he was too afraid he would be attacked by someone else, and had to be armed in order to protect himself. The examination ended at that point, and I recused myself from any further involvement in that case. I do not know what harm came to the examinee for not completing the examination, but I was relieved that at least no harm had come to me.

On another occasion, I warned a defense attorney not to go into a closed cell with his client, who had threatened to kill his attorney. The attorney disregarded my warning, went into the cell with his client and was able to be rescued by the guard, who heard his screams for help when he was attacked by his client.

Thus, harm in a forensic examination may be to the examinee, the examiner, or an attorney, or even the judge. The primary thesis of this book is to minimize or eliminate the harm that can occur to the examinee. Out of completeness, I felt it necessary to include others as well.

An example of avoiding or minimizing harm to an examinee can also result in minimizing harm to the examiner. Take, for example, a borderline female patient who has accused her psychiatrist of sexually abusing her. She has filed suit against her psychiatrist for boundary violation. The issue here is not whether the psychiatrist violated boundaries, but rather the best means by which such an individual can be examined without undue harm either to the examinee or to the mental health examiner. In such cases, I always insist on having the plaintiff's attorney present or a female "chaperone" present in the room to avoid any further accusations by the borderline patient who may perceive questions or comments or actions by the examiner as being offensive and boundary violations. Even though there is no doctor-patient relationship, the examiner is still expected to conduct the examination in a professional, non-harmful manner. Having a witness present accomplishes a number of positive results:

1. It allows the examinee to have a degree of comfort knowing that she is not alone with another psychiatrist whom she may fear will assault her or violate boundaries.
2. It allows the examiner the comfort to know that any inappropriate or false accusations made by the examinee against the mental health professional would be effectively rebutted by the witness in the office. Even though some colleagues feel constrained by having others present during such examinations, I welcome it as a means of protection not only for the examinee, but also for my own protection.

An example of what could happen without proper precaution or without an honest chaperone is the following:

I had been asked to examine for the defense a woman who had claimed that she had been sexually abused by her psychiatrist. She was clearly a borderline individual who had a history of making similar accusations against others. Fortunately for me, her attorney insisted that she have a special chaperone attend my examination. That chaperone was my former mentor and teacher of forensic psychiatry. I was pleased and delighted, because I knew that he was honest and that he would be a good witness in the event that I was falsely accused.

I had spent several hours with this individual who continued to turn to my former mentor in a pleasant manner, and to me with biting sarcasm and hostility. She had perceived me as the enemy and, as a borderline personality disorder, she perceived the world in extremes, either black or white, with no shades of gray. My mentor clearly was her champion, and I was perceived as her enemy.

Following the examination, I prepared a report, and the matter went to trial. At trial, the plaintiff accused me of improper questioning, improper advances toward her, including suggestive comments and inappropriate touching of her person during the examination. Of course, none of that had occurred, as she was malingering, or lying, or making this up, according to her own perceptions. Fortunately, my mentor and friend was honest in his testimony, indicating that his former student had been nothing but professional and that I had not conducted any of the boundary violations or professional errors of which I had been accused by this particular examinee. The plaintiff was shown to be an unreliable witness and lost her case because of her exaggerations and her false accusations.

What about videotaping or audiotaping the examination? I have no problem with either side or both sides taping my examination. In fact, it offers a degree of protection in case there are accusations of inappropriate comments, questions or behaviors, since everything is recorded. It offers protection for the examiner as well as the examinee.

What I do object to is audiotaping secretly the examination and then springing the tape on the expert in cross-examination at court without letting him know that the examination was taped and there is a transcript of that tape recording. My own experience with taping an examination is that the tape is usually not clear, it is not audible, and usually not very helpful or useful. Attorneys will alert the mental health professional that they want to videotape or audiotape the examination, and I usually agree as long as they are responsible for the taping and will provide me with the transcript of it before utilizing it in cross-examination in court.

4.15 Harm during Forensic Examinations

When considering the possible harm that could come to an examinee during a forensic psychiatric examination, the following 10 situations are relevant.

- examination of children or adolescents.
- examination of plaintiffs by defense experts.
- examination of criminal defendants by prosecution experts (especially in death penalty cases).
- the situation in which multiple examinations are required.
- the consideration of privacy or confidentiality when conducting assessments and obtaining as much information as necessary.
- the examination of a child who accuses an adult of sexual or other abuse, especially when the child needs to confront his/her abuser.
- the examination of women who claim to have been harassed or discriminated against at work and the detail in which they must relate their experiences.
- the examination of professionals for competency to practice their profession when their licenses may be in jeopardy.
- the evaluation and examination of a man accused of a sexual offense who may be considered a "sexually violent predator" (SVP) under the current legislation.
- the examination of the mentally retarded, the elderly, or the severely mentally ill.

4.16 Liability of the Forensic Examiner

Is the forensic psychiatric examiner liable for harm if the examiner is negligent in conducting the examination or if harm comes to the examinee as a result of the actions or omission of acts of the examiner? What recourse do examinees have if they feel they have been harmed during such a forensic examination?

Some colleagues have had negative experiences and have resorted to video-taping every forensic psychiatric examination in order to record the information and preclude lawsuits based on false accusations. Others have resorted to written agreements between lawyers and examiners about the liability issues, and have also had examinees sign agreements that the examination is conducted as part of a legal matter, that there is no doctor-patient relationship and no therapeutic requirements. Nevertheless, overt negligence may lead to damage and a lawsuit on rare occasions. What protections can forensic examiners take to avoid harm, not only to their examinee, but to themselves in a lawsuit at a later date? Many of these questions are addressed in the last two chapters of this book.

The best way to protect oneself and the examinee is to conduct the examination in an ethical manner following AAPL guidelines, striving for objectivity, seeking truth and justice, and showing respect for the examinee. Minimizing harm to the individual during the examination, report writing, and testimony is the best defense the examiner can utilize in preventing future lawsuits.

However, as there is no doctor-patient relationship, this is relatively uncharted territory with respect to malpractice lawsuits. Clearly, if the examiner conducts the examination with clear bias, hostility, and boundary violations, with intent to harm, the examinee may file a lawsuit, not on malpractice considerations, but on assault and battery or negligent professional behavior with intentional harm. Thus, minimizing or eliminating harm to the examinee during the forensic psychiatric assessment is not only beneficial to the examinee, but may also be helpful in preventing harm to the forensic expert.

References

1. Simon, R.I. and Wettstein, R.M. (1997) Toward the development of guidelines for the conduct of forensic psychiatric examinations. *Journal of the American Academy of Psychiatry and the Law*, **25**, 17–30.
2. Gutheil, T.G. and Bursztajn, H. (1986) Clinicians' guidelines for assessing and presenting subtle forms of patient incompetence in legal settings. *The American Journal of Psychiatry*, **143**(8), 1020–23.
3. Simon, R.I. (1998) The credible forensic psychiatric evaluation in multiple chemical sensitivity litigation. *Journal of the American Academy of Psychiatry and the Law*, **26**, 361–74.
4. Gold, L.H. (1998) Addressing bias in the forensic assessment of sexual harassment claims. *Journal of the American Academy of Psychiatry and the Law*, **26**, 563–78.
5. Appelbaum, P.S. (1997) A theory of ethics for forensic psychiatry. *Journal of the American Academy of Psychiatry and the Law*, **25**, 233–47.
6. Simon, R.I. (1996) Three's a crowd: the presence of third parties during the forensic psychiatric examination. *Journal of Psychiatry and Law*, **24**, 3–25.
7. Zonana, H. (1996) Ask the experts. *Newsletter American Academy of Psychiatry and the Law*, **21**, 16–17.
8. Stone, A.A. (1984) The ethical boundaries of forensic psychiatry: a view from the ivory tower. *Bulletin of the American Academy of Psychiatry and the Law*, **12**, 209–201.
9. Dattilio, F.M., Commons, M.M.L., Adams, K.M. *et al.* (2006) A pilot rasch scaling of lawyers' perceptions of expert bias. *Journal of the American Academy of Psychiatry and the Law*, **34**, 482–91.
10. (a) Perlin, M.L. (2000) *The Hidden Prejudice: Mental Disability on Trial*, The American Psychological Association Press, Washington, DC; (b) Perlin, M.L. (1989) *Mental Disability Law: Civil and Criminal*, vol. 3, Michie, Charlottesville.

5 The Forensic Psychiatric Report

Robert L. Sadoff

University of Pennsylvania School of Medicine, Philadelphia, USA

5.1 Introduction

There are very few articles written about how to write a good forensic psychiatric report. Simon and Wettstein have written on "the conduct of forensic psychiatric examinations," [1] and there are guidelines for psychiatric evaluation for Social Security Disability claimants [2]. Many articles have been written on conducting oneself as an expert witness in court, but very few on report writing [3].

A notable exception is a chapter by Robert Wettstein in the *Textbook of Forensic Psychiatry* edited by Simon and Gold [4], in which he states, "After completing the forensic evaluation, the evaluator is usually asked to prepare a detailed, written report of the evaluation. The evaluator should not, however, prepare a written report unless specifically requested to do so."

The forensic expert needs to assess whether he or she has sufficient data in order to prepare a meaningful report. Lawyers most often wish to have the expert call to discuss the matter before putting anything on paper. Some attorneys request a draft report, which the lawyer will then review and make recommendations for modifications or changes. Some attorneys may need or wish to have only a summary report to give as little information to the other side as possible while still giving the bottom line diagnosis and medical-legal conclusions or opinions. Others want a more detailed report that might include citations or references to support the conclusions reached. Most attorneys request something in between that is not so detailed, but also a report with more "meat" than just the bare bones.

Ethical Issues in Forensic Psychiatry: Minimizing Harm by Robert L. Sadoff
© 2011 John Wiley & Sons, Ltd

With respect to writing forensic psychiatric reports, Donald Hayes Russell [5] indicates there are four types of reports in criminal cases, each related to a particular phase of the legal process:

1. The trial examination report is a simple psychiatric assessment. Its purpose is to establish the defendant's legal sanity and competence, and the defendant is examined at the request of the court before he is put on trial.
2. The presentence examination report is made after the defendant has been found guilty and when the court asks advice of the mental health professional as to the type of sentence or disposition that is recommended.
3. Psychiatric follow-up reports may be asked for by the court whenever the court wants to learn what progress the patient is making.
4. Special reports are made if requested by the probation officer.

Wettstein states, "In general, the written report of the forensic evaluation must be comprehensive, detailed, precise, clearly written, and well substantiated. The purpose of the report is to communicate the evaluator's conclusions and supporting data to the retaining party and ultimately to the trial court or jury. The evaluator should assume that every word of the report is meaningful and exposes the evaluator to testimony on direct or cross-examination" [6].

Whatever the length of the report, it is important to consider the content. Because attorneys work in the adversarial system of justice, they oppose each other and attempt to argue as effectively as they can within the guidelines and regulations of the system. Attorneys may impose such adversarial extremism on the expert witness requesting the report to be written in as effective a manner as is consistent with the issues involved in the case. For example, the defense attorney, in a civil case, may believe the plaintiff is exaggerating his/her claims or is malingering about the extent of damage caused by the incident or the accident in question. The attorney may wish the mental health expert preparing the report to arrive at a similar conclusion and express it as clearly as possible in their report. Thus, attorneys may request changes in the wording of a report in order to meet their adversarial needs.

In my opinion, it is not appropriate for an expert to change their substantive opinion in order to meet the request of the retaining attorney. Some mental health experts will accede to the requests of the attorney to stay in good grace with the law firm that has retained them in order to be available for further cases in the future. (Unfortunately, some mental health experts see forensic work as a business rather than a profession and maintain their practice in a business-like way.)

Wettstein states, "Though the report should be focused around the referral forensic issue, related or even extraneous information about the evaluee is often appropriately included in the report, though retaining attorneys may not initially comprehend the justification for doing so. The evaluator must use judgment in deciding what is essential and relevant to include in the report. The evaluators can be questioned in court regarding why some information is included or not included in the report" [6].

It is permissible and ethical for the expert to modify his or her report by changing facts that are incorrect or by adding relevant or eliminating irrelevant material. However, removing relevant information such as preconditions that affect current diagnosis would not be appropriate or ethical.

As an example, plaintiffs' attorneys have requested that I not include prior medical history as it may confuse the issue of whether a particular incident was responsible for current mental symptoms. Sometimes, prior illnesses or prior medical conditions impact on a person's current mental state and are in part responsible for current symptomatology. Often, current mental conditions are multifactored and not related exclusively, or even substantially, to the incident in question that the plaintiff's attorney wishes to blame for his client's current mental symptoms.

5.1.1 Case Examples

A clear example is the case of a young woman who made the claim that she was sexually harassed and abused at work. Her history includes having been sexually molested by an uncle when she was eight years of age. She had received limited psychotherapy at that time and seemed to respond well without further symptomatology. However, following sexual abuse at work, she had symptoms that were serious and kept her from working. The plaintiff's attorney did not want to include the prior sexual abuse experience, because he was concerned that it would confuse the issue of workplace harassment and sexual battery causing her current symptoms.

The defense attorney wanted to emphasize the prior history, because he felt it was a substantial cause of her current symptoms rather than the incident at work. The answer is usually a combination of both. Clearly, the prior sexual abuse was significant in her life and added to the difficulties she experienced following the alleged workplace abuse. She was more vulnerable to the sexual abuse at work because of the prior experience with her uncle. That experience, of course, was significant and relevant, and added to her problems as one has to "take the victim as one finds her."

In a criminal case, a defense attorney requested that I not put information in my report about the defendant's family. The defendant was charged with a homicide during the course of a robbery. He has three brothers, all of whom are incarcerated on charges of armed robbery and drug abuse. The attorney felt this information would be inflammatory and prejudice the trier of fact. It was my belief that the information was relevant and must be included in the history. These facts may tend to harm the defendant in his criminal case, but they cannot be omitted as they are relevant, illustrating the environment from which he emerged and its impact on him and his behavior.

In another case involving a victim of violent sexual abuse, the perpetrator had raped and mutilated a middle-age woman whom he did not know and had met on the street. The attorney for the defendant wanted information in the report about the victim that included her prior use of illegal drugs, her having worked as a prostitute when she was younger, and her having been incarcerated on several occasions for petty theft and drug charges as well as prostitution. In some way, he had hoped by demeaning her, he would devalue her in the eyes of the jury so his client would not be seen as harming a regular human being, but one who was already "damaged goods." It was my opinion that the history of the victim was available to the trier of fact and did not need to be in my report, which focused on the defendant, his history, and his mental state. I did not need to harm the victim further by demeaning her in my report.

Wettstein recommends that the evaluator "maintain his ethical responsibility to strive for objectivity and, therefore, he needs to explore and consider all data sources rather than ignoring or even neglecting to explore the data that failed to support the expert's diagnoses and his opinions" [7].

5.2   Harmful Reports

It is the information contained in the report that can be damaging or harmful to people caught up in the adversarial system of justice, whether it be in a civil or a criminal matter. Consistent with the theme of this book, report writers should also attempt to minimize harm to the individual by carefully choosing their words. The defendant examined may be guilty and the plaintiff, in a civil case, may be malingering. However, it is for the court to determine the final verdict of guilt or malingering. The expert has a role in aiding the court in making a determination, but not being the final arbiter or judge of the situation. If the defendant, in a criminal case, indeed committed the crime and has no significant mental illness to aid in his or her defense, the expert for the prosecution may say so directly without casting aspersions on the "monstrosity" of the act or on the horrendous nature of the criminal behavior as, unfortunately, I have seen too often in some prosecution expert reports.

Also, if the plaintiff is malingering, as happens not infrequently, the expert for the defense may present the evidence to support such a conclusion rather than calling the plaintiff names such as "liar" or "deceptive." Unfortunately, too often the expert becomes entangled in the adversarial process and joins the attorney's wish to win the case. The expert witness should have no interest in the outcome of the case, but should remain, or strive to remain, as neutral and objective as possible.

5.2.1   Case Example

In one case that I examined, a young woman complained that she had been raped by her attorney when she sought help from him as a plaintiff in a civil action. It was learned in the course of the examination that she had five pregnancies. The first occurred when she was raped when she was 18, and she decided to keep the baby. She said she raised the baby as a single parent. The second pregnancy occurred when she was dating a man who impregnated her. She feared she would lose the fetus spontaneously when she began bleeding, but had a therapeutic abortion. The third pregnancy occurred when she was having an affair during the time that she was married, and did not tell her husband. She was careless, became pregnant, and had an abortion. The fourth pregnancy occurred with her husband and resulted in the birth of their son. Her fifth pregnancy was again during the course of an affair, and she had another abortion.

The attorney called, and asked that none of the information that he saw in my draft be included in the final report, because it would tend to put his client in a negative light, since she was suing for damages following a rape. I told the lawyer the information had to be included, because it was relevant and went to the damages that she sustained. The lawyer asked whether the information could be modified to show that for the second pregnancy, she knew she was losing the baby, and had the abortion only to stop the bleeding. The attorney also asked whether I could hold off the information that the third pregnancy was due to her having an affair while she was married and just say that she was careless and became pregnant, not indicating by whom the pregnancy was caused. I suggested that I could modify the way the wording was given, but that the information had to be in the report, because it was likely the other side had the same information, or would get it, and would wonder why my report was not as clear as it should have been. That would then go to the credibility of my opinion, which would negatively affect the plaintiff in court.

We decided, after a further discussion, to include all the information, but the matter would be worded in a way that would be less harmful or embarrassing to the plaintiff and still have full disclosure of the information. Clearly, the plaintiff was negatively affected by the rape by her attorney, and continued to have symptoms of PTSD, all of which were related to the instant offense and not to any of the prior pregnancies. I felt what the lawyer was asking was reasonable from the attorney's perspective, but not from the expert witness perspective, nor did I think it would negatively impact on the impression created by the report following the rape and the illness that she sustained as a result of the rape and the damages that she incurred.

5.3   Malingering

In one particular case, a woman complaining that she had been injured at work from harassment and a toxic work environment, came to my office on a warm day, dressed in several layers of clothing, supporting herself with two crutches, and refused to remove any clothing in my office. She spoke in an unusual manner, with inconsistencies, and it was clear that she was malingering. However, instead of calling her a liar, I suggested the defense attorneys obtain evidence of her malingering by videotaping her behavior at home when she was unaware that she was being observed. They did so, and found her dancing in the street with her daughter, without her crutches, in regular clothing, on a rather cool day. Her appearance in my office was a sham. My report recommending such observation declared that she is either the "sickest woman I have ever seen," or that she is malingering or exaggerating her symptoms in order to obtain an award from the court. It was clear that the latter was true, but I could word it in such a way as not to be harmful or adversarial.

In another similar case, a woman was left alone, unfortunately, by her attorney while I was testifying about her mental state to a mediator in the privacy of his office. When a nice looking young man walked up and asked her what she was doing there by herself, her response was unguarded, and she said, "I'm waiting for that shrink to finish his testimony after I had conned him in his office. He was examining me for damages, but there are none. I think I'm gonna get a lot of money on this case." She did not know the man had a microphone in his tie clip, which was connected to a tape recorder that he then took into the mediator, played for him, and the woman, of course, lost her case. In that instance, I did not have to malign the woman, as she did a better job of doing it to herself.

5.4   Ethical Issues

These are very difficult matters, because there are usually two sides to every question, especially in the adversarial system of justice. The defendant may be guilty of the crime charged, but may have mitigating factors, or even aggravating factors that could be relevant at trial. The plaintiff may have a valid complaint, but may also have had a predisposition for which the defense is not responsible. That is why it is so important for the expert to adhere to the ethical rules in forensic psychiatry, namely, seeking truth and justice and maintaining respect for the individual. Even though the credo is not "First, do no harm," the ethical position should be to at least minimize harm to the person caught up in the judicial system. The system itself can be stressful and harmful to both plaintiffs and defendants in civil cases, and to defendants in criminal cases. One may argue that defendants in criminal cases brought it on themselves to be in the position where they may be harmed by the system, whereas plaintiffs may have been innocent victims of a traumatic experience, through no fault of their own. Should one then have more sympathy for the plaintiff than for the defendant in a criminal case? Are all plaintiffs necessarily "innocent victims," or are some malingerers who are attempting to gain improperly from the system?

Consider, for example, the classic case of the SEPTA[1] bus in Philadelphia that left the terminal empty and crashed within a block of the terminal. Several people claimed they were injured on the bus even though it was empty at the time. They were looking to get something for nothing from the system. No sympathy for them, but one does not need to go out of one's way to brand them as criminals; in a sense, however, what they were doing was committing fraud and they may be charged criminally as well as being dismissed from the civil lawsuit.

One means by which the forensic examiner can maintain neutrality and objectivity is to stay within his or her expertise. We are not the attorneys who need to argue in an adversarial system. We are experts advising attorneys so they may argue with some scientific or professional support for their position. We may

---

[1] Southeastern Pennsylvania Transportation Authority.

advocate for our professional opinion and support it as best we can, but we are not adversarial in arguing a case. We must leave that to the attorneys and provide them with the information or evidence they can present to support their case.

5.5   Report Writing

With respect to the report, we must take a complete history and must include both positive and negative data that arise in the course of the examination. It is not fair to leave out the negative and only include the positive if one is working for the defense in a criminal case, or for the plaintiff in a civil case. One must include all aspects that are relevant.

However, in a recent case, the attorney asked that I not put in the report what the defendant said about his position with respect to the shooting of the victim. He had been accused by his three codefendants of being the shooter, and he had denied it. His stance was that he was present at the time and knew who did the shooting, but he was not "a snitch" and was not going to tell who the shooter was despite the fact that others had labeled him as the one who had done the killing. The attorney asked that I leave that to the prosecution to find and for cross-examination, if it came up at trial. The defense attorney has an ethical position to defend his client as zealously as possible. The prosecutor, on the other hand, is obliged to seek truth and justice, and not just win at any cost. Thus, the defense attorney has a right to tailor his expert's report so as not to aid and abet the prosecution. On the other hand, the prosecutor must include everything, even if it is negative to the prosecution's case, because it is relevant and it may lead to an acquittal.

Wettstein declares, "Perhaps the most significant deficiency in forensic mental health expert reports is the failure to adequately substantiate the evaluator's forensic opinions . . . Expert opinions without foundation are of limited value to the legal system . . . and need to be reached with reasonable medical certainty . . . [or] testimony will not be admissible in court" [8].

5.6   Trauma in Civil Cases

In civil cases, plaintiffs must put forward the reasons for their complaint and for the damages that can be supported by medical examination. They must also be able to show a link between the damages and the trauma of which they complain. That is, they must be able to show that what damage they have sustained was caused by the accident or the incident in question. Many symptoms may be caused by a number of different factors. We know, for example, that trauma does not cause schizophrenia or bipolar disorder, but it could certainly aggravate the symptoms the plaintiff had at the time of the incident.

Some attorneys have asked that I not include prior mental illness or treatment for other conditions, because it would dilute the effectiveness of the argument that the trauma at issue caused the illness in this case. I responded that could not be done, because it would not be fair to the defense not to include all relevant treatment and conditions the plaintiff had prior to this accident. It may even strengthen the plaintiff's case, because the prior incidents may have rendered him or her more vulnerable to damage from this accident that may not have been as damaging to a person not so vulnerable or so predisposed from previous similar trauma.

5.7   Case of a Harmful Report

In criminal cases, where violence is a factor, I often ask the defendant the triad of childhood firesetting, cruelty to animals, and late bedwetting, which often correlate with poor impulse control and later violent behavior. I have added a fourth factor of frequent fights in school, where either the individual had been the victim of bullying or was him- or herself a bully in school.

One particular defendant in a homicide case had bragged about the number of fires he set as a child and how they had stimulated him to further firesetting. He also admitted that he had wet the bed until the age of 11, and was brutally beaten each time by his mother or father for that behavior. With respect to cruelty to animals, he was very proud of the fact that he had killed a number of cats in a brutal and vicious manner and had also shot birds and dogs with his b-b gun, first blinding them and then cutting them up after they were staggering around. He seemed to enjoy relating that he did this and was pleased with his behavior. I included that in the report for the prosecution, indicating that these were behaviors that correlated with the violence of the crime for which he had been charged.

The defendant was furious that these details were in the report, because he felt they harmed him and even though they were true, he did not feel they should have been included as they put him "in a bad light." It is true that they do tend to put him in a bad light as a violent person who is proud of and pleased with his violent behavior, but they are facts that I felt needed to be included in the report and would not remove them. Were they harmful to the defendant? Of course they were, but without them, I would not have had a complete report. Here I did not minimize the harm to the defendant, but these were not the kind of data that could be omitted, even though they were harmful. As I indicated, we cannot always eliminate harm, but we can attempt to minimize it whenever possible.

5.8   Civil Case Report

In a recent civil case in which a woman complained that she had been traumatized at work and suffered damage due to age, gender, and racial discrimination, I had seen her as suffering from PTSD from the extreme stress of her work-related conditions, which were clearly outlined in the report. The defense had two psychiatric expert reports, but did not compare them before sending the reports, written separately and independently by the two experts, to the plaintiff's attorney. One had done a comprehensive evaluation of the woman and reached the conclusion that she was malingering, that these behaviors never occurred at work, and that she had nothing wrong with her and should not be compensated for her perfidy. The other expert reached the conclusion that she had had a prior condition of bipolar disorder that did not relate to the conditions at work; even though she was extremely mentally ill, according to his assessment, the illness preceded her work, was not caused by it, and she should not be compensated for it. Both denied that she had any symptoms of PTSD.

The matter was resolved in court when the defendants settled, because they knew the experts would contradict each other and their case would be significantly weakened. The woman clearly had symptoms of PTSD, was not bipolar, and was not malingering. However, experts may differ in their assessment and look at different parts "of the elephant in the middle of the room," and come to different conclusions. Reaching different conclusions is acceptable in forensic psychiatry, depending on the data on which the conclusions are based. However, submitting reports that are so opposite, that harms the case, is not acceptable and should not have occurred.

In another case, a psychiatrist conducted an MMPI[2] that did not comport with his conclusions. In his report, he dismissed the MMPI as sometimes not being valid and not always being accurate. In my opinion, he should have not included the MMPI at all, because it harmed his conclusions and actually supported mine as the expert on the other side. In court, I was ready to attack his conclusions and utilize his MMPI results to support my own opinion. However, before I could comment on his report, there was a sidebar conference, and I was instructed not to comment on him or his report at all since he would not be called to testify.

It should be noted that I am against psychiatrists utilizing psychological tests that they have not been trained to administer, to score, or to interpret, but rather administering only one of many that is scored by computer and then using the results either to bolster their opinion or not using it at all. I think it brings harm to the profession to use instruments that one is not properly trained to utilize. Psychologists spend years learning to administer, score and interpret tests, and to utilize a battery of tests correlating data from one test to another, rather than just relying on one self-administered test.

5.9 Content of Reports

We should utilize, in our reports, words that we wish to convey opinions about, and to omit any extraneous comments, words, phrases, sentences that either are not relevant or are superfluous. We should write the reports in clear English, leaving out professional jargon whenever possible. Ideally, there should be subheadings and means to ease the way of reading the report. I do not always label a paragraph "Mental Status Examination," but clearly, the content is the mental status of the examinee. I have been criticized in others' reports, rebutting my report, that I did not even have a mental status examination or that I did not utilize a *DSM-IV-TR* [9] diagnosis in my report. I have since learned to label my paragraphs so that even the worst readers will know that the paragraph contains the mental status examination. I also attempt to utilize *DSM-IV* diagnoses whenever possible, and where relevant.

---

[2] Minnesota Multiphasic Personality Inventory.

Another example of avoiding harm in the report is to avoid including information about a person that is harmful, embarrassing, and not relevant to the case. For example, I examined a woman who was charged with shoplifting, and in the course of the examination, she told me about five abortions that she had had, even though she had been raised Catholic and had a moral conviction against having abortions. She also stated that she was bisexual and had several different lovers of both genders. She also was a cross-dresser, and had some serious sexual problems that were not relevant to the shoplifting.

I recognize that sometimes sexual problems are related to shoplifting, but in this case, they were not, and it was better for her to plead guilty to the minor offense than to have her whole sexual life, which was embarrassing to her and to her partners, revealed in court.

There was a particular issue, however, that needed to be reported, and that was that she was thinking about taking her life and also taking the lives of several of her lovers. She had recently purchased guns which needed to be put in safekeeping. She was in therapy, and with her permission, I contacted her therapist and told her about the confessions to harm others and herself, and with the help of the therapist, we were able to put the guns in safekeeping and put the young woman in a hospital for treatment so she would not be harmed and would not harm others.

The issue here is minimizing harm in the report. The embarrassing sexual material did not need to be in the report, but the violent behavior that she anticipated did need to be; that was reported, and she was properly treated.

5.10 Using Harmful Words

In writing reports, the use of particular words may be misleading, confusing, harmful, or adversarial. For example, instead of saying, "Mr. Jones denies any sexual diseases such as HIV, AIDS, syphilis, or gonorrhea," it may be better to say that "there is no history of Mr. Jones having such illnesses." Also using the words, "denies use of drugs or alcohol" may be read differently from the words that Mr. Jones "states he has not abused alcohol or drugs." The implication of the use of the word "denies" is that denial may be untruthful.

The use of the word "malingering" may be pejorative, and it may also be speculative. One should probably avoid using words such as "malingering" unless it is in the form of a *DSM-IV-TR* diagnosis, with proper numbering and evidentiary support for it. Similarly, words such as "lying" and "deceptive" should also be avoided. Perhaps, it is best to say the person seemed inconsistent in his or her revelations, and then give examples of the inconsistency. Are these inconsistencies unconscious, or is there a conscious motive to deceive?

Also, in the report, it is best for the examiner to utilize such words as "If what the person tells me is true, then these are my opinions." However, too many plaintiffs' experts will accept the words of the plaintiff as being factual, and on the basis of those "facts" will render an opinion as though the "facts" were absolutely "true." I have suggested that we word our reports in the subjunctive rather than the declarative mode, such as—"If what the plaintiff tells me is true, then she does have PTSD from the alleged assault on her at the workplace by her supervisor." We do not know that the supervisor attacked her, and the supervisor, in his sworn deposition, has denied such an attack. We have only the plaintiff's word for it, even though that also was sworn under oath to be factual. Again, it is a matter of not taking sides in the adversarial system, but trying to strive for objectivity and neutrality as much as possible.

5.11   Attorney-Expert Relationship

Elsewhere, I have written: "Psychiatrists should discuss with retaining attorneys their preferences regarding a written report. Some cases will not require a written report. Others may require extensive reports."

"Psychiatrists should send the proposed report to the retaining attorney only and not to anyone else. Attorneys can then decide to whom they wish to forward copies of the report ... and assume both responsibility and liability for any consequences that come from disseminating the information" [10].

An example of the kind of adversarial position that psychiatrists can take occurred in a fairly prominent murder case where one man killed his friend "for no reason at all." The prosecution had no motive for the killing, and the defense, therefore, jumped on the concept that the defendant must have been insane when he did the killing, because there was a finding of mental illness in the defendant. The prosecution expert, finding a minor mental condition not consistent with psychosis, opined that the killing occurred under the influence of alcohol and drugs. There are psychiatric experts who tend to find alcohol and/or drugs as the basis for violent behavior in many cases, and ascribe the behavior in question to substance abuse.

The issue of the expert being an independent agent and not an agent of the attorney who pays his fees, is important. It is permissible for psychiatrists and psychologists to consult with attorneys and to make modifications in factual errors in their reports, but not the conclusions they draw, unless warranted by professional observations and opinions. Too often, attorneys try to influence their experts to word their reports and present their testimony in such a manner that is consistent with their extreme adversarial position. There are times when experts should argue effectively with the retaining attorney regarding various concepts and wording in their report and not permit such intrusions on their professional independence. It is perfectly proper for attorneys to refuse to call their experts to testify if the experts cannot accommodate them with a report that supports their adversarial position. In such cases, I have convinced attorneys that it would be better for them to present their case without my testimony, inasmuch as the essential consideration in expert testimony is credibility.

In a particular case, the attorney wished to plead his client not guilty by reason of insanity. This was a young man who had a diagnosis of bipolar disorder, and when he became manic, he became violent. During one of his manic episodes, he shot and killed two people whom he believed had betrayed him. At the time he did the shooting, he knew that he was killing them and intended to do so. He understood what he did, and knew that it was against the law for him to shoot them, even though he believed they were betraying him. He was clearly seriously mentally ill and needed to be in treatment. He also required confinement in a secure environment in order to prevent further violent behavior. On the surface, it appeared as though this man was also legally insane. However, on close examination, it was clear that he did know what he was doing and knew that it was wrong, but did have difficulty in conforming his conduct to the requirements of law. In Pennsylvania, that becomes "guilty but mentally ill" rather than insanity. I convinced the attorney to present the case in that light in order to get a reasonable sentence for his client, because pleading him insane would not have succeeded, and he would have received either two life sentences or the death penalty.

Another case demonstrates the importance of working with the attorney in order to avoid harm to the defendant. A young woman in her twenties had solicited a man to kill her father. During the time she was waiting for the homicide to occur, she changed her mind, "backed out at the last minute," and told the prospective killer not to carry out the assignment. For some reason, he ignored her pleas to save her father's life, and did kill her father. She was arrested as a coconspirator and was charged with first degree murder. She was clearly seriously ill and traumatically stressed due to the sexual and physical abuse she had experienced at the hands of her father (which was the reason she wanted him dead). Nevertheless, she was not psychotic, was not mentally retarded, and was not so severely battered by her father that a jury would decide that he deserved punishment of death. It was my opinion that she should plead with extenuating circumstances. A negotiation was accomplished whereby she would receive three years in prison as an accomplice.

While waiting for the negotiation to be completed, she was convinced by another psychiatrist to not accept the plea and to plead not guilty by reason of insanity, and that psychiatrist would testify for her. The reports were submitted, and it was clear that she was not insane, and the other psychiatrist suggesting insanity did not do her a service. In fact, she was harmed by the suggestion that she plead insanity. She was found guilty, and sentenced to 25 years in state prison instead of three years on a negotiated plea. I am certain the other psychiatrist was convinced, in his own mind, that he was doing the right thing and was helping the defendant. But, as stated earlier, "Sometimes with the intent of doing good, we cause more harm." I have found, in the practice of forensic psychiatry, that a team approach is best, where the expert works closely with the attorney in order to accomplish a successful conclusion. When there is a distinct difference of opinion, it is the client or patient who often suffers.

5.12   Recommendations in Reports

I have reviewed reports in which forensic psychiatrists have recommended not only long term incarceration in a maximum security environment be given to this person (presumably as punishment), but in some cases, have indicated in their reports that "no treatment would be helpful to this person, and punishment is the only recourse." Putting such a statement in a psychiatric report, in my opinion, goes too far. The mental health expert should put in the report that either psychiatric treatment will be helpful or there should be reasons given why treatment is not warranted or is not likely to be helpful to this particular individual. For example, if the defendant charged in a brutal homicide case has had repeated offenses despite treatment that had never been effective, certainly that would be an appropriate comment to include in the report. However, if this were the first offense, it is not proper, in my opinion, for a forensic psychiatrist to put in the report that this is a "repeat offender." I have seen in some reports by mental health experts for the prosecution in sexual offender cases, that the person is a repetitive sexually violent person where the statute required more than one sexual offense to warrant such a label being utilized. When there is only one offense and not repeat sexual offenses, I think that labeling a defendant a repeat sexual offender is uncalled for, is biased, prejudicial, and takes the extreme position of the prosecution rather than "striving for independence, objectivity, or neutrality."

Similarly, I have seen cases in which there was an incident of one non-violent sexual offense, such as exhibitionism or voyeurism, or a minor touching in a case of frotteurism. For some reason, the evaluator for the prosecution saw fit to include in her report a statement that this was a repetitive behavior and the perpetrator deserved to be labeled a sexually violent predator (SVP). The examiner testified, under cross-examination, that she made that statement because even though there was only one incident in which the individual was arrested, clearly, he must have committed this offense several times since it is the kind of crime that people do more than once. I believe that is not a fair statement, is speculative, and is not based on scientific evidence.

Wettstein presents a table of potential problems or errors found in forensic report writing [8]. Included in his list of 15 items are the following of importance:

- failing to consider all data sources in reaching opinions.
- mixing data and expert opinions.
- suppressing disconfirming data.
- relying on unsubstantiated diagnosis and expert opinions.
- addressing the wrong forensic issue.
- allowing attorney-requested changes in an expert's opinion.
- submitting inaccurate curriculum vitae.

Further, he states, "The evaluator must remain within his or her expertise, use accepted rather than idiosyncratic psychiatric theories, correctly interpret the professional literature, use the data extant in the case and not fabricate information." "Evaluators should be open to changing their diagnosis and expert opinion upon the receipt of additional information."

5.12.1 Case Example

There was a plaintiff in a civil suit, a Mr. M., who alleged he developed PTSD as a result of a motor vehicle accident (MVA). Dr. J., who was retained to examine Mr. M., reported to the attorney that although Mr. M. did have PTSD, his disorder was causally related to a traumatic assault that occurred earlier that year.

The doctor believed that his current symptoms were exacerbated by the MVA, but not caused by the MVA.

Mr. M. had not told his attorney about the earlier trauma. When the attorney originally consulted Dr. J. about the case, Dr. J. stated that she believed the proximate causation could be demonstrated. However, because the attorney did not know about the earlier trauma, she could not tell the doctor about it, not until the evaluation was completed and the information became available. When the attorney read the expert report, she was very upset with Dr. J. because she could not use it to demonstrate proximate cause, which jeopardized winning a large settlement in the case. She had considered the case "open and shut." So the attorney asked the doctor to delete the information regarding the earlier trauma and change the opinion to reflect that Mr. M's symptoms were causally related to the MVA. Dr. J. felt she could not ethically provide a report regarding the causation of PTSD that did not include the information that the plaintiff suffered a prior trauma that had caused the symptoms in question. She advised Ms. B. that she could not make the requested change [11].

Problematic requests for changes may also include leaving out essential or relevant data that is harmful to the examinee. Changes that remove essential data are also not appropriate. Certain facts may not be relevant, depending on the purpose of the report and so could be deleted without altering the nature of the opinion. For example, in a criminal case, the jury does not need to know about prior criminal acts. If the report is to be admitted into evidence, the psychiatrist may leave out the information about previous criminal charges or convictions. However, in the sentencing phase of the trial, the information about the prior criminal case is relevant and should be included.

Lawyers may also request changes in opinions when the opinions must be formulated without the benefit of a personal examination of the evaluee. Such circumstances can arise in cases involving wills and testamentary capacity, suicide or criminal matters when defendants refuse to cooperate with examinations. Attorneys often like to have a diagnosis for a variety of reasons. Psychiatrists should be very cautious in giving a diagnostic impression without having examined the individual. They can indicate that the symptoms noted in the records are consistent with a particular diagnosis, but they should refrain from giving a declarative diagnosis even when a lawyer may request such a definitive response.

Some attorneys ask to review a preliminary draft before the final report is issued. If drafts are prepared, they should be kept and not discarded. Psychiatrists who choose to prepare a draft should be prepared, on cross-examination, to acknowledge this and to produce the preliminary drafts. Failure to provide the drafts can result in the presumption on the part of the cross-examining attorney, and perhaps even the court or the jury, that the psychiatrist was attempting to conceal changes made in original opinions to suit the retaining attorney. However, some forensic psychiatrists routinely discard all previous draft reports and indicate this is their usual practice in all cases.

5.13   A Final Caution

Even though the examinee is told at the beginning of the examination that there can be no traditional doctor-patient confidentiality and that whatever the patient says in the course of the examination will be put into notes and perhaps in the report, during the examination there are times when the examinee will ask to say something "off the record," or does not wish to have the information put in the report. Examiners may be curious about what examinees have to say, but really cannot guarantee that anything is "off the record." If they hear it in the course of the examination, they may have to report it, and should not agree that they will listen to it, put their pen down, turn off the tape recorder, and not report it. That would not be honest or fair.

5.14   Assessing Physicians' Fitness

It is especially difficult at times for psychiatric experts to assess a physician's fitness for duty when it is challenged because of drug addiction, alcoholism, sexual boundary violations, or other mental health problems that may impair or impede the physician's ability to function. Anfang [12] and others refer to the American Psychiatric Association's research document on guidelines for psychiatric fitness-for-duty evaluations of physicians and state, "The evaluator should offer an opinion about whether the physician suffers from a psychiatric illness; whether that illness, if present, interferes with the physician's ability to practice safely in his particular job; and the specific reasons and areas of impairment, including insight and judgment ... The focus is on the psychiatric impairment and assessments of unsafe medical practice."

Further, the authors note the written report on such fitness-for-duty evaluation should include the concept; "If no impairment is found, the data should also be articulated with a clear logical explanation that substantiates the conclusions. The report should not just briefly conclude that there is no problem and therefore the physician is fit for duty" [12].

These authors are referring to the preparation of a report that if not properly done could be harmful to the physician who is examined. The authors note there are a number of factors that could affect decisions about what information to include in the examiner's report. They note that in general, the smaller or more local the referral source, the more likely that medical and other personal information will be viewed by individuals who personally know or may have conflicts of interest with the physician being evaluated. In order to avoid embarrassment or harm in such a local situation, the authors recommend that the examiner might "state that she collected detailed information about personal, medical, and social history that substantiated her opinions, and that she can provide a more detailed report of that data on request" [12]. It is important in all cases, however, that specific positive or negative findings about fitness for duty be well explained and substantiated in the report.

The authors are also concerned about the examining psychiatrist in such cases. They state, "Psychiatrists who contemplate conducting these evaluations may be concerned about their own liability risk. An unfavorable outcome or a medical error resulting in patients being harmed by a physician who has been recently found fit for duty could result in allegations of malpractice or negligence against the examining psychiatrist" [12].

Psychiatrists recognize that in such evaluations there is no treatment relationship established that could possibly preclude successful malpractice claims. However, allegations of negligent evaluations can still be made, even if they are successfully defended. The authors recommend the examiner present "a thoroughly documented report, including any limitations and uncertainty of the opinion due to incomplete, inaccurate, or missing data" [12].

In assessing individuals for Social Security Disability, there are guidelines for such determination, and lack of knowledge of these guidelines could lead to harm to the claimant, because the evaluator would not be knowledgeable of the standards to be met in the assessment and the examination. The authors of the article note that "a poorly written report may delay or prevent award of appropriate benefits," thereby harming the claimant. It may also "prejudice later determination of the claimant's appeal." The written report becomes part of the claimant's SSA[3] record, which will be reviewed if the case is appealed or at the time of continuing disability investigations. Thus, in this particular situation, the report in Social Security Disability is extremely important and, if poorly done, can cause harm to the claimant.

5.15   Summary

This chapter is not a treatise on how to write a report, or how to conduct a forensic examination, or how to testify in court. Others have written more eloquently on those subjects [3,4]. This is a treatise on minimizing harm in the examination, the report writing, and in testifying in forensic cases. The harm may be to the examinee, to the examiner, or to the attorney. If one can eliminate, prevent, or minimize harm to any of those three entities, the purpose of this treatise will have been successful.

References

1. Simon, R.I. and Wettstein, R.M. (1997) Toward the development of guidelines for the conduct of forensic psychiatric examination. *Journal of the American Psychiatry and the Law*, **25**, 17–30.
2. Folsom, J., Lipsett M., Raskin, D. *et al.* (1983) Committee on rehabilitation of the American Psychiatric Association, Guidelines for psychiatric evaluation of Social Security Disability claimants. *Hospital and Community Psychiatry*, **34**, 1044–51.
3. (a) Gutheil, T.G. (1998) *The Psychiatrist in Court: A Survival Guide*, American Psychiatric Press, Washington, DC; (b) Gutheil, T.G. (1998) *The Psychiatrist as Expert*

---

[3] US Social Security Administration.

Witness, American Psychiatric Press, Washington, DC; (c) Rappeport, J.R. (1992) Effective courtroom testimony. *Psychiatric Quarterly*, **63**, 303–17; (d) Simon, R.I. (2005) Standard of care testimony: best practices or reasonable care? *Journal of the American Academy of Psychiatry and the Law*, **33**, 8–11.

4. Wettstein, R.M. (2004) The forensic examination and report, in *Textbook of Forensic Psychiatry*, (eds. R.I. Simon and L. Gold), American Psychiatric Press, Washington, DC, pp. 139–64.

5. Russell, D.H. (1971) The Court and the Expert: Writing Reports, Vol. 1: Writing Reports for the Massachusetts Courts. *International Journal of Offender Therapy*, **1**, 14–19.

6. See Ref. [4], p. 155.

7. See Ref. [4], p. 158.

8. See Ref. [4], p.156.

9. DSM-IV-TR (2000) *Diagnostic and Statistical Manual of Mental Disorders*, 4th edn, Text Revision, American Psychiatric Press, Washington, DC.

10. Sadoff, R.L. (2004) Working with attorneys, in *Textbook of Forensic Psychiatry* (eds. R.I. Simon and L.H. Gold), American Psychiatric Press, Washington, DC, pp. 165–82.

11. See Ref. [11], p. 173.

12. Anfang, S.A., Faulkner, L., Fromson, J. and Gendel, M.H. (2005) The American Psychiatric Association's resource document on guidelines for psychiatric fitness-for-duty evaluations of physicians. *Journal of the American Academy of Psychiatry and the Law*, **33**, 85–8.

6 Expert Psychiatric Testimony

Robert L. Sadoff

University of Pennsylvania School of Medicine, Philadelphia, USA

6.1 Forensic Testimony

Following a comprehensive forensic psychiatric examination and the preparation of a forensic psychiatric report, the psychiatrist is sometimes called to testify about the opinions given in the report, either at deposition and/or at trial in court. Hoge and Grisso [1] comment on the role of the forensic psychiatric expert in court: "The proper role (of the expert) is to describe the relevant abilities, disabilities, symptoms, and diagnostic conditions in clinical and behavioral terms, leaving to the court to weigh these observations in the context of legal concepts and standards."

The purpose of this chapter is not to present the techniques that exist for psychiatrists who testify, but rather to discuss ways of minimizing harm that can occur during testimony. Harm may come to the defendant in a criminal case, the plaintiff or the defendant in a civil case, or to the expert witness, to the attorney, or to the judge in a criminal or civil matter.

6.2 Danger to Attorneys

In criminal cases, the defendant may be excessively violent, and during the course of the examination of the defendant, a threat may have been made to harm the defendant's attorney. I have warned attorneys to be cautious of clients who have threatened to harm them because of paranoid delusions that the attorney is working in conjunction with the prosecution to conspire to have them found guilty and send them to prison. I have also alerted attorneys that their clients are out to harm them and they should not be alone with them. I have alerted female attorneys that their clients are potentially sexually violent toward them, and they should be cautious when alone with the defendant in his cell.

Ethical Issues in Forensic Psychiatry: Minimizing Harm   by Robert L. Sadoff
© 2011 John Wiley & Sons, Ltd

6.3 Danger in the Courtroom

Occasionally, there is an outburst by the criminal defendant in court that has harmed people in the courtroom. Consider, for example, the case of the man in Atlanta[1] who grabbed a sheriff's gun and shot and killed several people before he was apprehended.

Consider also the man in Minneapolis [2] who had secreted a razor blade in his boot from the jail and, while sitting at counsel table listening to the testimony of the woman he had abducted and raped, that she did not love him as he had believed in his erotomanic delusion, leaped over counsel table, grabbed the razor blade from his shoe, and slashed her face while she sat helpless on the witness stand. There was no way to prevent that violence, because it was neither predictable nor foreseeable, except that he had protested the day before from counsel table that she did love him.

6.4 Harm to Expert Witness

Harm may come to the expert witness who is cross-examined on personal material that is irrelevant, but may be allowed by the judge. Experts have been asked personal questions about their private lives [3], their divorces, their sexual lives, especially if they are testifying in a case involving sexual abuse, or a contested divorce. The rationale is that the attorney is looking for bias if it exists.

6.5 Attacking the Expert in Court

In discussing the potential harm to the expert witness, one must consider impeachment techniques by skilled attorneys during cross-examination. Goldstein [4], an attorney-psychiatrist, states, "Attacks on the credibility of the psychiatric expert witness are termed impeachment. This article provides an in-depth review of the various impeachment techniques used by lawyers during cross-examination and offers specific suggestions to the psychiatric expert witness on how to prepare for and counter some of these trial ploys."

Goldstein distinguishes between substantive evidence and credibility evidence. Attorneys may ask expert witnesses whether they testify for one side exclusively, or whether they are available to both sides in either civil or criminal cases. Another issue is the amount of money experts receive for their work. Is it based on their testimony or on their time? Do they charge for the whole day if their testimony only takes one hour? Goldstein suggests the forensic psychiatrist "should be involved in a wide range of professional activities such as teaching, private practice, or hospital work. Such activities not only enhance professional skills, but tend to refute allegations that the psychiatrist functions as a full-time expert witness" [4].

---

[1] *State v. Nichols*, in which the defendant, Brian Nichols, shot and killed a judge and was sentenced, on December 13, 2008, to life imprisonment with no possibility of parole for four murders of which he was convicted. There are no court decisions from an appeal in this matter.

Goldstein also alludes to statements experts have made in prior cases that may be inconsistent with their testimony in the instant case. He states, "The more an expert witness testifies, the more likely he is to have a record of saying something that may be opposite to what he is saying in this particular case" [4]. He gives the example of the prediction of future violent behavior, the expert may testify in a particular case that one cannot tell or that it is very difficult to tell, or one needs special testing or information that was not available in that case. In the current case, however, the expert may be testifying that the person clearly represents a danger to self and others and this may be refuted or challenged by his prior statement.

Goldstein discusses "persecution" of the expert witness, that is, improper use of impeachment techniques. He states, "A number of cases indicate that at times lawyers are carried away by their zealous advocacy during a trial: From time to time it has come to pass trial lawyers have occasionally acquiesced to their baser instincts and refer to the opposing witness in terms less than becoming the decorum of the courtroom" [4]. Goldstein cites a case in which the prosecutor, in his summation concerning two of the defense psychiatrists, specifically referring to them as "the two happiness boys, those two idiots—I'm sorry, those two psychiatrists." He "charged" them with being "ignorant stupid incompetent," and scoffed at their titles of "diplomate." He notes these remarks were improper and cannot be justified or excused by anything that transpired earlier in the trial. He also notes that in another case the Appellate Court censured the prosecutor for repeatedly resorting to ridicule and sarcasm in order to impeach the credibility of the defense psychiatric expert witness. Goldstein concludes, "Although courts condemn such inexcusable and improper remarks directed at expert witnesses, they usually regard them as merely 'technical error,' that is, not depriving the defendant of a fair trial or warranting a reversal" [4].

I have been asked in court to comment on cross-examination whether I respected my adversary psychiatrist in a case tried before a judge without a jury. The judge overruled the objection by my retaining attorney and said, "I want to hear what Dr. Sadoff has to say about Dr. X." My response was that, "I respect Dr. X's right to disagree with me." That, of course, is not the answer he was seeking, but the judge understood the implication and did not pursue it any further.

In another case, the expert witness for the other side criticized my treatment of a particular defendant in a criminal case, suggesting that psychoanalytically oriented psychotherapy was totally inappropriate and the defendant should have had cognitive therapy from the beginning. He was brutal in his criticism of me as a therapist. He made the mistake of staying in the courtroom to listen to my testimony. When I agreed that he should be the therapist and give cognitive therapy and did not badmouth him in any way, he came to me after the testimony and apologized profusely for his verbal outburst. I told him the lesson that he learned from this experience was never to badmouth a colleague in court.

The opposite occurred in a case in which I praised my adversary because he was worthy of praise; it was surprising to him. We had been on the opposite sides of a criminal case in a southern state where I testified for the defense and he, a very prominent elderly psychiatrist, was called by the prosecution to rebut my testimony. He was an expert on hypnosis who had published widely and extensively on the subject. He was well known internationally and well respected in his field. When I was asked, on cross-examination, whether I knew him, I said, of course I knew him—everybody knows him. He was world renowned, well respected in the field of hypnosis. The case, of course, was not about hypnosis, but about dissociative identity disorder (DID). When we broke for lunch, he stopped me and asked why I praised him so highly. "Aren't we supposed to be on the opposite sides of this case?" The doctor was not a forensic psychiatrist and did not understand that even though we are in an adversarial situation, we can disagree without being disagreeable and he was deserving of the praise.

There are many times when I have been asked about the reputation of my colleague on the other side of the case. Usually, I know the other expert and praise him or her when praise is due. I indicate that we have a disagreement on this particular case, but on other cases we have worked together and we have agreed. I find that juries like this open and honest approach and the lack of rancor or hostility. Juries do not like when psychiatrists battle each other or when lawyers viciously attack the expert psychiatrist.

Thus, in addition to avoiding harm to the examinee, that is, the plaintiff or the defendant, experts should also avoid harm to themselves, their profession and, clearly, to their adversary.

6.6   Harm to the Defendant or Plaintiff

All of this is to say that the courtroom can be a dangerous place for witnesses, bystanders, participants, expert witnesses, and claimants or defendants. Primarily, the concern is for the defendant in a criminal case or the plaintiff, in a civil case. Questions may be asked that can lead to very damaging testimony that can harm the individual. Sometimes that cannot be avoided, because the defendant, in the criminal case, is truly a psychopath or has a diagnosis of antisocial personality disorder and requires punishment and confinement. However, there are cases in which expert witnesses may not fully understand the implications of the mental illness or diagnosis and testify inappropriately.

6.6.1   Case Example

In one case, a woman had expressed concern about harming her baby after her daughter was born. She received psychotherapy and medication, and did very well. She was advised not to get pregnant for five years; and she did not. She raised her daughter without difficulty, and then did become pregnant when her daughter was five years of age. She was counseled by her therapist during her pregnancy so that she would not have a similar postpartum depression, and she would receive medication after delivering her child. Her son was born; she was placed on antidepressants, and seemed to do well. However, after a month, she was left alone with her son when her husband took their daughter for lunch. The son disappeared, and it turned out that she had a dissociative event that led to dropping the son in a nearby river, leading to his death by drowning. She had no memory of the event, but under hypnosis, was able to discuss the killing of her child and other self-destructive experiences she had during pregnancy. She sought punishment for herself due to her belief that she had been guilty of various behaviors that were based more on fantasy than reality.

Initially, she was going to receive two and a half to five years by the judge for involuntary manslaughter. However, after a comprehensive evaluation by a forensic psychiatrist, there was a full blown hearing on a guilty plea, with efforts to show that she had suffered from a postpartum psychosis due to hormonal imbalances, and that the death of her infant was directly related to and caused by her postpartum psychosis, with dissociative events. A non-physician expert, a psychologist with presumably no training in medical hormonal imbalances, testified that the judge should put her away for a longer period of time, until her daughter was old enough to protect herself from her mother's potential violence. (She had never been violent to her daughter.) The judge accepted the psychologist's view, and sentenced her to 8–20 years in state prison, until her daughter was 13 or 14 and could defend herself from her mother, though there was never any threat against the daughter and the hormonal imbalance that caused her violent behavior to her son had passed when she stabilized (as people do after having postpartum illnesses).

The judge clearly was misled by the psychologist, who did not understand the nature of the defendant's illness and testified sincerely about his view of her condition, wishing to protect the life of her daughter. However, he did so with erroneous belief that she posed a danger of harm to her daughter when, in fact, she was never a danger to her and took care of her daughter for five years without difficulty, having never threatened her daughter in any way.

It is this kind of testimony, based on inaccurate information, if not professional ignorance, that can be harmful to people. Expert witnesses have a certain amount of power that must not be abused or misused to the detriment of others' freedom or their lives.

6.7   Standards for Experts

It is for these reasons that courts have established standards for testimony, including Daubert [5] and Kumho [6] that limit the testimony of expert witnesses to scientific conclusions rather than "junk science" that too often invades the courtroom. Judges can serve as gatekeepers to keep such testimony out if they are sophisticated enough to know the difference.

The old Frye [7] test of 1923 limited the testimony to that which has been accepted by a majority or a significant minority of professionals working in the field. Some states continue to utilize Frye, but others have adopted Daubert, which mandates that the testimony not only be scientifically based, but also be of help to the jury or the fact finder in making judicial decisions.

In the article on "Peer review of psychiatric expert testimony," the American Psychiatric Association's Council on Psychiatry and the Law [8] approved the conclusions of the Committee on Peer Review of Expert Testimony. The Committee noted that in general, informed criticism of courtroom testimony by psychiatrists falls into two categories: "Judges, scholars, and legal and psychiatric practitioners have criticized the competence of some psychiatrists who testify in court. The most frequent complaints heard are that psychiatrists may fail to understand the legal issues at stake, to have a firm enough grounding in the relevant empirical literature to be able to draw scientifically well founded conclusions, or to communicate their findings and opinions understandably to judge and jury" [8].

The second group of objections to psychiatric testimony relates to the ethics of courtroom testimony. Critics complain, for example, that some psychiatrists "deliberately distort their testimony to serve the interests of the people who are paying them, or to advance other causes to which they are sympathetic" [8]. This critique calls into question the dedication of some psychiatrists to the concept of truthfulness in court.

The Council suggests remedies for these two objections. "One is educating the expert, and the other is sanctions by the organizations for violating ethical norms" [8]. The Committee made decisions about standards that could be applied to review of expert testimony. The Council did not attempt to develop written standards for forensic testimony. They found their absence was not an impediment to the peer review process. They did suggest the formulation of general standards or principles for experts' conduct would be desirable.

Five years later, there was an analysis and commentary on the American Psychiatric Association Resource Document on Peer Review of Expert Testimony in the *Journal of AAPL*, 1997 [9]. The Council suggested the following distinct functions for the psychiatric expert following four different roles:

1. the psychiatrist as expert on scientific knowledge.
2. the psychiatrist as expert on medical practice.
3. the psychiatrist as expert on the mental condition and behavior of particular individuals.
4. the psychiatrist as expert advisor.

These four roles are appropriate for the psychiatrist testifying in court. None of them involves the psychiatrist as adversary, but primarily as a teacher sharing scientific knowledge, information about medical practice, and observations of mental conditions and behavior of particular individuals within the justice system. The psychiatrist, as expert advisor, again is as a teacher sharing information with the jury or the fact finder that they would not be expected to know. By maintaining a role as teacher and advisor, the mental health expert in court minimizes harm or damage. He or she does so by not assuming the role of adversary arguing their case, but rather sharing information as a teacher would to students. By maintaining these "professorial" or academic roles, the expert witness not only minimizes harm to the subjects involved, but also minimizes harm to the profession of forensic psychiatry and to the experts themselves.

6.8   Exaggeration

Expert witnesses may also be harmed by their own testimony or exaggeration of their credentials. Some experts have inflated their curriculum vitae and indicate that they are "board eligible" for their board certification in psychiatry or forensic psychiatry. Board eligible means that a person has completed the requirements in order to take the board examination. The lawyer should always ask whether: The examination was taken? Was it passed? Or had it been failed? And how many times has the expert taken the exam? Sometimes, individuals with a master's degree refer to themselves as psychologists and, in some areas, the psychologist must have a PhD in order to be so labeled. When experts are caught exaggerating their credentials or misinforming the court about the number of publications or their training or experience, they cause harm to themselves and their clients, because their credibility is in question.

An example of such testimony that was effectively rebutted was the statement that I had made on direct testimony in a homicide case that I had evaluated in 45 years of work, over 10 000 people charged with crime and over 3000 charged with homicide. The prosecutor began his cross-examination by challenging my numbers, believing that I had inflated the number of cases I had examined. He began by stating very clearly that I had said, on direct examination, that I had examined over 10 000 people charged with crimes. I acknowledged that was true. He said, "Let's do the math." I said, in response, "Alright, let's do the math." He challenged my numbers by saying that there are about 250 workdays per year (five days a week for 50 weeks) so that I would have to see one person a day for 40 years to reach the 10 000 mark. I assured him that I had seen more than one per day for several years and that I had been counting not only the private cases, but also the ones that I saw as a consultant at various hospitals and forensic psychiatric hospitals at which I consulted on a regular basis. When he realized that the math was in my favor and that I was not exaggerating the numbers, he went on to another topic for cross-examination.

The message here is that one can give as accurate an estimate of one's work as possible, but one should not overestimate. I have seen people who have testified that they have examined many more than 10 000 people and they worked only 10 or 15 years, and it would be almost impossible for them to have seen that many people in so short a period of time. So the response would be, "Let's do the math." That holds for other comments made by the expert witness about his or her experiences. In today's world of computers and Google, there is no privacy. People can determine from the computer what one's experience has been and can even determine which cases a person has evaluated and testified.

Another way experts can harm themselves is through testimony that is not based on accepted scientific principles or on direct experience. When an expert testified that an individual had paranoid schizophrenia and was asked, under cross-examination, how the expert determined that diagnosis, the response was, "I'm a psychiatrist. It's a gut feeling, I know." That also diminishes the expert's credibility, as it is not an acceptable response.

Very few experts have been charged with perjury or direct lying under oath in court, but some have been accused of puffery or exaggeration. One individual testified that he had directly examined the plaintiff for three hours when, in fact, the record shows that it was only 45 minutes. Another testified that he had spent four hours at the prison examining a defendant when the sign-in book showed that he had been there for only one and a half hours and had to wait half an hour before seeing the defendant.

6.9   Unusual—Unscientific Testimony

Another expert testified that the defendant could not have known what he was doing, because he was acting with a 15-month-old brain when he killed another man. The expert was asked about that statement, and said that the defendant had a sister who was born when he was 15 months old and his brain stopped maturing at that time. Thus, he was left with a 15-month-old brain and he could not be held responsible for his behavior. The judge admonished the expert, telling him that he did not really have to say that, because it was incredible and unbelievable, and the jury would have difficulty with it. Nevertheless, he persisted.

Another expert witness embellished his credentials by indicating that he was a student of one of the great forensic psychiatrists in the country. The teacher acknowledged that the young man attended a one-hour lecture course that he had given at a national meeting, but that he had not spent any other time with him and could not be considered his student. Again, that kind of embellishment hurts experts and their credibility, not to mention the effect it has on their clients, who are the ultimate losers.

6.10   Malingering and Inconsistent Opinions

Perhaps, the most egregious type of harm that occurs in testimony is a direct verbal assault on the plaintiff in a civil matter, or on the defendant in a criminal case. In one civil case, the plaintiff had complained that she had been the victim of sexual and racial harassment at work. One expert examined her, testified that she was a direct malingerer, that is, that she was lying about what happened and lying about her symptoms. Another expert, who did not check with the first one, testified that she had a serious mental illness that preceded her work history and her symptoms were not as a result of any work-related trauma or harassment. During testimony, the expert who labeled her a malingerer was confronted with the report of his colleague and flat out said that his colleague was wrong, that she did not have any mental illness, and that she was an out-and-out liar malingering her symptoms. The other psychiatrist, who had labeled her as having a major depressive disorder that preceded her work, testified that she was not a malingerer, that she did have bona fide symptoms, but they were not related to her work history.

The plaintiff's expert, who had received all the records from work as well as statements of others who observed the harassment and testified that it was real and not fantasized, and also had treatment notes from her therapist, who had treated her for several years, indicated that she did have a depressive disorder that preceded her work, but she also had symptoms consistent with PTSD that were caused by the work-related trauma and harassment.

The credibility factor favored the plaintiff, primarily because of the total disagreement between the two defense experts, but also because the plaintiff's expert based his testimony on the records and the testimony of others who supported his contention, his diagnosis, and his conclusions.

6.11 Attorney-Expert Relationship

Sometimes, experts want to please the retaining attorney and testify according to what they believe the attorney wishes to hear or to have the expert testify in court. This attitude and expectation can lead to a lack of credibility on the part of the expert witness.

I had the unhappy experience of examining a criminal defendant, finding that he had serious emotional problems, and gave the opinion that he had a diminished capacity at the time of the commission of the act in question. I so indicated in my report and in deposition testimony. By the time we got to court and I testified, I was asked, on cross-examination, various questions that had not been asked previously, questions that seriously affected the testimony that I had previously given, requiring me, for credibility, to modify my opinion based on the new facts that I had not previously received from the defense attorneys.

I had received a check prior to my testimony, which is my requirement in order to enter the courtroom. When I tried to cash the check, I found the check had been canceled, and I tried to question the attorney, who would not respond to my phone calls or letters. He finally did respond to my attorney, telling him that he canceled payment on the check because he felt that I had changed my testimony that harmed his client, and it was not in keeping with the testimony I had given at deposition or that I had in my report. When I reviewed my previous testimony and my report, I found that, in fact, the testimony was similar, but had to be modified in order to be credible with the new evidence. Since his client was found guilty, he felt that he could not pay for the expert testimony and did what I would consider to be unethical for an attorney and, that is, to stop payment on his check. That was the one and only time that has ever happened. He could not have been sincere about my testimony, because a few years later, he called again requesting me to examine another of his clients. I refused to do so when I recognized who he was and that I could not trust him. The lesson here is preparation and obtaining all new records that may affect testimony before entering the courtroom.

6.12 Preparation

There was another time when I testified in a criminal case before a judge, without a jury, and did not have all the records, because the lawyer had no time to prepare my testimony before I went on the witness stand. I had testified in favor of the defendant until, on cross-examination, a document was shown to me that indicated that I was wrong and the document would change my opinion. When

I so testified, the defense attorney jumped up, saying, "But I showed you that document." I said, "No, you had not, and if you had shown it to me, I would not be here today testifying for your client." Needless to say, we have never worked together again, and his client was harmed, because he failed to show me all of the documents, including the ones that were harmful to his client. It is important for attorneys to know that they must have total disclosure of documents to their experts if the expert is going to help them in court. Clearly, one cannot hide such documents that will be produced on cross-examination and will only hurt the defendant. It was my opinion that this was an oversight by the defense attorney, who has a reputation for being an excellent attorney.

6.13   Controversial Testimony

I recently had the experience of waiting to testify in court about a defendant's competency. This 60-year-old man had been diagnosed as having bipolar disorder for the past 35 years and had been seen by eight different mental health professionals all of whom diagnosed him as having bipolar disorder. He was sent for evaluation to a federal hospital where he was examined for over a month by a psychologist who concluded that he did not have bipolar disorder and that he "merely had a mixed personality disorder." The doctor found that he was competent, because he was manipulative and knew the participants in the courtroom and their functions. She believed that he could work with his attorney if he chose, but because of his personality difficulties, he chose not to be cooperative. She had never met the attorney and had not had an observation of the dyadic relationship between the two of them. It was my opinion that she sincerely believed in her testimony that the defendant did not have bipolar disorder in spite of the fact that psychological testing, on two different occasions by two different psychologists, confirmed the diagnosis. One psychologist indicated that the testing was also consistent with cyclothymic disorder as well as bipolar disorder. She chose to focus on that aspect of it rather than the bipolarity.

The issue here was not whether the defendant understood his position within the legal system, as he was extremely bright and could certainly know who the participants in the courtroom were and their functions. What kept him from being competent was his bipolar disorder that prevented him from working rationally with his attorney in preparing his defense. He would not listen to him, he would call reporters and the press and make statements that were harmful to him and his case, and he would give information on several different topics at the same time in a loose association with a flight of ideas.

Clearly, he required treatment in a hospital with medication that he had taken before that had been helpful to him in order to restore his competency so he could be tried. In my opinion, it was harmful to him for a prosecution expert to deny the existence of a psychotic illness with which he had been diagnosed for several years by many different mental health professionals. She also argued that when a label was given to a patient, it continued without consideration of the fact that it might be wrong from the beginning. That may be true if it were one or two times, but with eight different examiners at different times in different places giving him the same diagnosis, the question is, "Were they all wrong?" When asked, she acknowledged that they were all wrong and she was right. She is certainly entitled to her opinion, but fortunately for the defendant, the evidence of his serious psychotic mental illness was sufficient for the judge to find that he was incompetent to stand trial and required placement in a treatment setting.

6.14   Attorney Influences on Expert Witnesses

In addressing the influence attorneys have on expert witnesses, Slovenko [10], discusses the role of attorneys selecting experts and presenting their testimony in court. He states that it is the attorney's responsibility in presenting the mental health expert in court with reference to different elements of the trial process. He notes how the attorney goes about doing it, why it is necessary, and especially the relationship between the attorney and the expert witness in how the attorney may influence the testimony of the expert. He presents such issues as "fabrication of testimony, providing and withholding of data, motive presentation, sequestering witnesses, compelling expert testimony" and other matters that affect the mental health expert in court.

Slovenko notes the necessity of having expert witnesses in various cases contributes to the integrity of the judicial process. He states that as the adversary system evolved, experts hired by the parties gradually replaced court appointed experts who were found not to be without bias. "The nature of the adversarial process, to be sure, almost invariably forces the expert (once deciding to serve as a witness) to be aligned with the party who engages him, and in that sense, to be biased as well. He is, however, not presented as a neutral, as was the court appointed expert. This process has a built-in anti-abuse device—the cross-examination, a time-honored technique for testing competency or credibility" [10].

Slovenko notes that it is the duty of a lawyer "to employ, for the purpose of maintaining the causes confided to them, such means only as are consistent with truth and never to seek to mislead the judge or juries by any artifice or false statement of the law" [10]. He shows, as a part of a cartoon, an attorney saying to his expert, "Just remember that lying can get you into a lot of trouble if not done properly." Slovenko states, "The lawyer is ethically bound not to fabricate evidence. Preparation of the witness is good lawyering, but coaching of a witness is grounds for a reversal" [10].

6.15   Experts and Attorneys

Don Harper Mills, an attorney physician, states:

> No amount of written advice will help you if your lawyer is incompetent. He should be your shepherd. He should see that you prepared properly, look properly and act properly. He should help to calm the troubled waters, to steer you back when you deviate, to soften the sting of your misstatements. If he cannot or will not do these things, you are going to get nervous [11].

He declares, if that happens, the witness then "takes over." He refers to that as disaster and points out, "The expert is now the advocate; his credibility as an impartial expert is shot, and so is the lawsuit." He states, "If you feel you are stuck with an inept lawyer, either withdraw or see it through with dignity; then have nothing more to do with him" [11].

Jonas Rappeport [12] asks the questions on initial contact with the attorney regarding the anticipated questions and the cross-examination. He recommends the expert review the entire file, including depositions, "prepare, prepare, prepare." He states, "know the facts, know the dates involved in the cases." He notes that what is most important in court is the expert's "objectivity, professional experience, ability to explain concepts in lay terms, personal appearance as an expert witness in the judge's courtroom. What is least important to the judge or jury is possession of a law degree, membership in a professional organization, honors and awards, where trained, number of publications or journals and books" [12].

Gutheil and Simon [13] conclude, "While most attorneys practice ethically and treat their retained experts fairly, there are a few that do otherwise." The authors describe "early warning signs" of the likelihood that the attorneys' attempting to retain the psychiatric expert witness may compromise the expert's honesty and striving for objectivity. The authors refer to early warning signs which include the following:

1. assumed opinion by the expert;
2. selective data;
3. misinformation or deception about the insurance picture.

Danger signs for the expert include:

1. the vulnerability to attorney pressure;
2. the expert who is considered to be a "hired gun," giving whatever is asked of him or her by that side;
3. the desperate expert, that is, one who needs the money;
4. the new expert who wants more cases from that law firm;
5. the expert who "needs to be loved;"
6. the expert "on a mission."

The authors recommend overcoming some of these obstacles by having

- a clear and detailed fee agreement;
- one's consciousness raised by discussions, to note the blind spots regarding signals that may also stand the expert in good stead;
- regular consultation with colleagues about this lonely, often isolating work in which the attorney may be the only non-patient with whom the expert converses during the work day.

They suggest the expert should continue to "strive for freedom from bias that may emerge from any direction, including attorney pressures. Only in this manner can ethical practice be preserved" [13].

Goldstein [14] states, in his not so optimistic view that Gutheil and Simon have illuminated on this "critical aspect of forensic practice that has been neglected today, in providing the early warning system to guide the practitioner over this 'tricky terrain.'"

Stone [15] in discussing Simon and Gutheil, contends that Gutheil, who is busy, can turn down 20–30% of his cases, but a number of people cannot. Stone states, "Forensic psychiatry's allegiance to the ethos of honesty as opposed to the medical ethical ethos of *primum non nocere* (first of all, do no harm) is a clear recognition of the different contexts in which they serve and the adversarial challenges and pitfalls of the expert witness" [15].

Michael Dearington [16], an attorney, states that mostly attorneys and experts are competent and honorable and concludes, "Out of all of this background, the truth generally emerges, and justice prevails."

Hoge and Grisso state, "Mental health experts' clinical opinions do not have to answer the legal questions of competence or criminal responsibility in order to provide valid assistance to court. Their proper role is to describe the relevant abilities, disabilities, symptoms, and diagnostic conditions in clinical and behavioral terms, leaving to the court to weigh these observations in the context of legal concepts and standards" [17].

So how does the forensic expert minimize harm in testifying?

- The mental health expert must have all the information available in the case.
- The expert should prepare adequately and effectively with attorneys before entering the courtroom.
- The expert should stay within his or her area of expertise and not testify on issues that are beyond his or her ken or expertise.
- The expert should refrain from making damaging statements not based on fact or scientific evidence.
- The expert should not badmouth a colleague on the other side of the case.
- The expert should be aware of any changes in the defendant or plaintiff in court that might lead to an eruption or violent behavior that may be anticipated and, therefore, prevented whenever possible.

6.16 Summary

Unfortunately, a number of forensic mental health experts become identified by their political position in various cases. There have been individuals who are known as prosecution experts or defense experts in criminal cases, or as defendants' experts or plaintiffs' experts in civil cases. It is important, in my opinion, for a person to be available to evaluate individuals for both sides so that one does not gain an identity as a person who is biased toward one position or the other. Clearly, any bias should be revealed in court under cross-examination with respect to questions such as: "How many cases have you done for the prosecution? How many for the defense? And, in how many cases that you saw for the prosecution have you found incompetency or insanity in the defendant, and vice versa, how many cases examined for the defendant have you found the person to be competent and not insane?"

These are important considerations, primarily from the standpoint that harm may be done not only to the person examined because of the inherent bias of one or both of the examiners, but harm may come to the profession because of the bias perceived on the part of the expert witnesses.

References

1. Hoge, S.K. and Grisso, T. (1992) Accuracy and expert testimony. *Bulletin of the American Academy of Psychiatry and the Law*, **20**, 67–76.
2. *State of Minnesota v. Ming Sen Shiue*, 326NW 2d 648, (Minn., 1982).
3. Gutheil, T. (1998) *The Psychiatrist in Court: A Survival Guide*, American Psychiatric Press, Washington, DC.
4. Goldstein, R.L. (1988) Psychiatrists in the hot seat: discrediting doctors by impeachment of their credibility. *Bulletin of the American Academy of Psychiatry and the Law*, **16**, 225–34.
5. *Daubert v. Merrell Dow Pharmaceuticals*, 509 US 579, (1993).
6. *Kumho Tire Co. v. Carmichael*, 526 US 137, (1999).
7. *Frye v. United States*, 293F 1013 (DC.Cir. 1923).
8. American Psychiatric Association's Council on Psychiatry and Law (1992) Peer review of psychiatric expert testimony. *Journal of the American Academy of Psychiatry and the Law*, **20**(3), 343–52.
9. American Psychiatric Association Resource Document on Peer Review of Expert Testimony (1997) *Journal of the American Academy of Psychiatry and the Law*, **25**(3), 359–69.
10. Slovenko, R. (1987) The lawyer and the forensic expert: boundaries of ethical practice. *Behavioral Sciences and the Law*, **5**(2), 119–47.
11. Mills, D.H. (1984) A review of testifying in court. *Journal of Forensic Sciences*, **29**, 587.
12. Rappeport, J.R. (1992) Effective courtroom testimony. *Psychiatric Quarterly*, **63**(4), 303–17.
13. Gutheil, T.G. and Simon, R.I. (1999) Attorneys' pressures on the expert witness: early warning signs of endangered honesty, objectivity, and fair compensation. *Journal of the American Academy of Psychiatry and the Law*, **27**(4), 546–53.
14. Goldstein, R.L. (1999) Commentary on attorneys' pressures on the expert witness. *Journal of the American Academy of Psychiatry and the Law*, **27**(4), 554–8.
15. Stone, A.A. (1999) The forensic psychiatrist as expert witness in malpractice cases. *Journal of the American Academy of Psychiatry and the Law*, **27**(3), 451–60.
16. Dearington, M. (1999) Commentary on attorneys' pressures on the expert witness. *Journal of the American Academy of Psychiatry and the Law*, **27**(4), 559–62.
17. See Ref. [1], pp. 73–4.

Part Three

Vulnerable Populations in the Justice System

7 Children and Adolescents

Robert L. Sadoff
University of Pennsylvania School of Medicine, Philadelphia, USA

7.1 Introduction

Perhaps two of the most vulnerable populations examined in forensic psychiatric matters are children and adolescents. A child may become a victim of sexual abuse or a victim of a physical trauma in a motor vehicle accident. Children may also be the victims in a battle between their parents or among adults regarding their custody or visitation privileges by either parent. In criminal cases, a child or adolescent may be charged with criminal behavior, most likely theft, shoplifting, drug possession or sales, or assault, and battery. Occasionally, a minor is charged with a serious felony such as murder or attempted murder.

The examination of children or any minor is a very special examination that requires sensitivity, experience, and training in child psychiatry as well as forensic psychiatry. Children who are victims of sexual abuse or incest are particularly vulnerable in forensic situations. They may have been threatened by their predator or assailant with death, or death of their parents if he or she tells of the abuse. They may be frightened that they will be killed if they speak to an examiner about what happened to them. Also, many children tend to repress the experience through dissociative techniques to protect their integrity. Many children have difficulty communicating with strange adults about innocent matters; needless to say, they will have great difficulty communicating traumatic experiences unless a skilled interviewer or examiner knows how to communicate effectively with the child.

Having been privy to the "family secret," the child may be unwilling or unable to discuss the traumatic experiences. Often, the child will want a trusted parent with him or her before meeting with the child forensic psychiatrist. How much of the traumatic experience must the child relive in discussing it with the examiner in order to satisfy a proper forensic child psychiatric assessment in such cases? How much harm do we have to bring to the child in order to accomplish our mission of conducting a thorough and complete assessment in seeking justice and truth? In these cases, there is a real balance of harm versus truth-seeking.

Consider the number of cases of domestic relations battles where fathers are falsely accused of sexually abusing their daughters in order for the mother to gain an advantage in the legal proceedings. Consider also the number of cases in which overzealous therapists have implanted memories of sexual abuse in their patients in order to arrive at what they consider to be "the truth" of the origin of various symptoms within their adult patients.

In keeping with the theme of the book of minimizing harm, a number of cases will be presented illustrating the need to balance the acquiring of information with the minimizing of harm to the child or adolescent in producing the necessary information in order to proceed effectively. Criminal cases against adult sexual perpetrators of children have been lost because of inadequate, ineffective, or poor interviewing of the children, which led to inadmissible testimony. Sometimes, it is tempting to lead the child to the conclusion the interviewer "knows" is true. However, all interviews of children in these cases should be videotaped in order to protect the rights, not only of the children, but also of the adult defendants who may not be guilty of the crime charged. Also, there have been cases where the perpetrator has been guilty, but could not be adjudicated as such in court because of faulty interviews with children who were the victims of sexual crimes. In those cases, harm is done to the system of justice, to the profession for inadequate or improper interviewing techniques and, clearly, to the victim who will not have judicial satisfaction after having been sexually abused and harmed. In essence, the child will be "doubly harmed" because of an improper judicial result.

In criminal cases where the child or adolescent is the defendant, harm can come if the child is not interviewed properly regarding motivation, involvement of others, and proper diagnosis. The law has established rules for police interrogation of minors, requiring an adult to be present during the minor's statement to the police.[1] I would recommend a similar proposal for mental health experts examining children who are defendants in criminal cases. I would recommend all such interviews be videotaped if an adult cannot be present. Even with an adult present, I would recommend the videotaping to document the examination. Did the interrogator lead the vulnerable minor to give statements that are not true, but may be expedient to relate under the circumstances? At other times, it is better not to have family members present; for example, when interviewing a 13- or

---

[1] In Pennsylvania, Statute 42 Pa. C.S. Section 6326 requires that the parent or guardian of the child being taken into custody be notified "with all reasonable speed and without first taking the child elsewhere." In federal law, the section is 18 U.S.C.S. Section 5033.

14-year-old female who has just been arrested for killing her newborn infant when the family was not even aware that she was pregnant.

The laws have changed in a number of states regarding decertification of minors charged with crimes. Some states, for example, Pennsylvania,[2] start the minor as an adult and have a hearing to decertify the defendant to be tried as a juvenile rather than as an adult. In neighboring New Jersey,[3] the procedure goes in the opposite direction, starting the minor as a juvenile and having a hearing to certify him or her as an adult, if appropriate.

In summary, children and adolescents involved in the legal system are more vulnerable to pressure, intimidation, and undue influence than more mature adults. Special precautions must be taken by examining forensic mental health experts when children and adolescents are involved. In civil cases, one has the problem of evaluating a youngster who has been physically and/or emotionally injured. The examiner must be familiar with developmental issues in children and how such trauma may impede their emotional as well as physical growth. What effects will the trauma have on the youngster as she develops into a young woman? For example, the problem of a facial injury that leads to severe scarring will have a more significant impact, in our culture, on females than it will generally on males. Also, the loss of limbs in budding young athletes due to injury will also have significant impact and effect upon the victims of such trauma. The hopes and dreams of a number of young people have been dashed because of injuries. That all needs to be recorded and compensated appropriately through careful evaluation and assessment of current damages, and also projecting damage into the future.

The impact of sexual abuse on young males may be as devastating as it is to young females. It is well known that males are less likely to report their having been sexually abused than are young females [1]. The shame and embarrassment is overwhelming for some who cannot tolerate the memory of the trauma.

In domestic relations battles, where perhaps most children are seen in a forensic context, the trauma can be highly significant, especially when the child is caught between the demands of a loving mother and a loving father. Children are often required to choose or to make decisions about preferences that they are not prepared to make. Sometimes, the role of the forensic child expert is to advise the court on how to proceed in terms of limiting the testimony of the child and not putting the child in the untenable position to make a decision that he or she is not prepared to make. Recommending whether the child testify directly facing his or her perpetrator is another matter for consideration. Often, judges will allow a screen between the child and the defendant who is accused of sexual abuse. Sometimes, the child can give testimony on videotape to the court to avoid a direct confrontation.

---

[2] Decertifying juveniles from adult to juvenile court is 42 Pa. C.S. Section 6322. The law in Pennsylvania certifying a juvenile from juvenile court to adult court is 42 Pa. C.S. Section 6355.
[3] NJ Statute Section 2A:4A-26.

7.2   The Role of the Child Forensic Psychiatrist

Haller [2], in describing the role of the child forensic psychiatrist, notes it is not fundamentally about avoiding harm or about how harm may occur to the child. Specifically, he states,

> *The forensic examiner's opinion may result in harm befalling the examinee. For example, a juvenile defendant faces waiver to adult court. If the examining child psychiatrist concludes that the youth is not a candidate for rehabilitation under the auspices of the juvenile court and the judge concurs, the child is tried as an adult. One might conclude that participating in the process, the psychiatrist is causing harm to the child [3].*

Haller also notes,

> *The forensic evaluation of a minor is inherently different from the traditional diagnostic evaluation. In the latter sense a minor is brought to the child psychiatrist for the purpose of alleviating suffering. A diagnosis is made, doctor-patient relationship is formed, and the examiner is bound by several medical, legal, and ethical principles. In contrast, the forensic child psychiatrist's role is to answer a legal question [3].*

Haller indicates that examples include custody, visitation, and parenting plans; whether the child has suffered emotional harm from an injury; or whether the child is competent to stand trial as a juvenile. He states, in these examples, "The psychiatrist is not acting in a traditional role in that no doctor-patient relationship is formed and the end product is different from a therapeutic relationship" [3].

Richard Ratner [4], a prominent child forensic psychiatrist states the Code of Ethics of the American Academy of Child and Adolescent Psychiatry (AACAP) is a third pillar on which the ethical practice of clinical child and adolescent psychiatry rests. "As physicians and psychiatrists, members are bound by both the AMA [American Medical Association] and APA guidelines. The AACAP code attempts to refine and clarify these principles because of the uniqueness of the child as patient" [4].

Enzer delineated three aspects of this uniqueness:

> *First, children are dependent but become more independent over time; second, children are uniquely vulnerable both because of their dependency and because of the 'potential for intimidation and coercion' by parents and others; and third, despite their vulnerabilities, children and adolescents remain 'individual human beings' and, as such are entitled to be taken seriously and respected [5].*

Ratner states further, "In common among all of these codes are the principles of beneficence and non-maleficence (to do no harm), from which exhortations to practice competently, show compassion and respect, be honest, safeguard confidentiality, and respect the law all derive." He concludes, "Even more care must be taken when dealing with a child or adolescent, because they are in varying degrees dependent and incapable of taking full responsibility for themselves" [4].

Ratner notes, "The aim of a forensic evaluation differs from the clinician's job of helping or caring for the patient. Furthermore, the forensic evaluator's primary allegiance is generally to a third party, whether it is the court or an attorney involved in an adversarial process" [4].

Because children and adolescents are presumed by society to be less than fully responsible for their actions, "they are seen both as needful of the support of competent parenting figures and, if having offended, the substitute parenting of the states … thus, it is critically important for any psychiatrist involved in the evaluation to act in a fully ethical way" [4].

Ratner states the types of evaluation generally performed (in forensic child psychiatry) are unique to this age group. "Custody and related matters, including relocation, termination of parental rights, parent evaluations in cases of abuse and neglect, and foster care and adoption, are the most common focus of involvement with younger children. Evaluations of suspected sexual abuse also fall within the forensic sphere. Evaluations related to juvenile justice are more common with older youth" [4].

He notes these will include evaluations for competency to stand trial, criminal responsibility, waiver or transfer to adult court, and evaluations of sexual offenders. He believes the most common focuses on the most appropriate disposition for the youthful offender [6].

Ratner emphasizes the ethical duties of the forensic child psychiatrist in custodial and juvenile criminal matters [6]. In summary, Ratner proposes that as long as the forensic child psychiatrist is aware of the ethical guidelines and practices in an ethical manner, the risk of harm to the children or adolescents involved in forensic matters will be minimized [6].

7.3   Domestic Relations Cases

In domestic relations disputes, there are often accusations made, some of which are accurate and truthful, and others are given for an advantage in the court and may not be based on fact, but rather on bias or prejudice. The forensic examiner should make every effort to sort out the veracity of such accusations whenever possible. Goldzband [7] has written of domestic relations matters as "the ugliest litigation." He points out the nasty accusations that are made by hurt parents when they feel betrayed or rejected. They will often lash out, and some will even hurt the children in order to get back at the other parent. How can we minimize harm in such extreme situations?

First, the examiner must understand the totality of the situation in which the child is involved. Second, the examiner must be aware of the forces impacting upon the child in these cases. Third, the examiner must be aware of the symptoms the child has shown since the breakup of his parents' marriage. Children will often regress and begin to wet the bed, have speech problems, school-related problems, behavior problems, temper tantrums, and even more serious psychological symptoms that resemble psychosis. Many will alienate themselves from one parent and attach to another, or withdraw within themselves and become depressed. Some will show symptoms of school phobia or agoraphobia, not wanting to leave home, where they feel more secure. Some older children will begin to act out by using drugs, skipping school, sexual promiscuity, and other self-destructive behaviors they would not ordinarily have engaged in absent the traumatic family situation. The examiner must be sensitive to the needs of the child and the fears and concerns of the child in this very difficult legal situation.

This is why I strongly recommend that a well-trained child forensic psychiatrist conduct these assessments, and not just anyone who has a degree that says "I'm able to do this." It takes experience, sensitivity, and a motivation to conduct a thorough ethical forensic examination while minimizing harm to the children involved.

The examiner must be aware of the concept of "parent alienation syndrome" developed by Gardner [8], in which one parent alienates the child or children from the other parent. There is much controversy about this concept, and it is not universally accepted. However, the examiner must consider the possibility that one parent is badmouthing the other to the children in order to gain a foothold in the legal proceedings.

Another concept is that of the children banding together in order to attempt to resolve the issues themselves. One case concerned five youngsters from the ages of 5 to 11 who were caught in the maelstrom of family disruption. Although they had been physically and emotionally abused by their mother, they chose to stay with her because they recognized that she was mentally ill and needed them more than their father did. They were willing to sacrifice their well-being in order to take care of their mother. They felt that father could get along without them or only with visitation, but they needed to be home with mother in order to take care of her. This was the concern of the 11-year-old boy who convinced the others that he was correct. It was my concern, as the forensic examiner, that the children would be harmed by the mother and that their concern for her, although altruistic, was not in their best interest. The matter was resolved by allowing the children to ventilate their concerns and their choices and to avoid further abuse by the mentally ill mother by making certain that she received proper treatment while visiting with them under supervision so they could maintain their concern for her without being harmed.

7.4　Best Interest of the Child

Miller cites a case that came before the United Supreme Court, *Palmor v. Sidoti*, (1984) [9], in which the Court made the decision on the legal best interest of the child, that was not in her psychological best interest. Miller declares the expert's role is not to become involved in the moral correctness of the court's decisions. He states, "the expertise of the psychiatrist is not in democratic principles; it is in the development of affective relationships. Unlike the Supreme Court, the psychiatrist cannot make judgments based on fairness to the mother" [10]. He notes that in this case the Supreme Court's judgment considered the equal protection of the mother, that is, her best interest. He concludes it did not consider the equal protection of the child. He further states, "Only the mental health worker is solely committed to the child's emotional best interests. All others have conflicting loyalties. The judge follows legal precedent. The attorneys represent the parents' wishes. The parents have to balance their welfare with that of their child" [11]. Miller closes with the following statement:

It is important for the expert to stick to the task, even if placed in an enormously uncomfortable position. The expert's opinion may bewilder the court. The parents may hate him. A good solution for the child, however, is an act of preventive psychiatry and is far more effective than psychiatric treatment afterward. Although the doctor carries an impossible burden, knowing that he or she has served the child's welfare is reward enough [12].

Miller clearly delineates the role of the child forensic psychiatrist in advocating for the best interest of the child irrespective of the rights or interests of other parties involved in this litigation. He notes the various roles of the judge and attorneys, but the specific role of the mental health expert is to advocate for the best interest of the child, that is, minimizing harm to the child in these very complicated and complex cases.

Thus, the child forensic assessor must be aware of the techniques, not only of conducting the interview or several interviews of the child, but also collateral interviews of significant others in the family, as well as joint interviews of the child with either parent and with both parents together when appropriate.

7.5 Child Abuse and Neglect

Barnum [13] suggests that there are four issues, some of which may not be explicitly raised in referral questions when mental health experts become involved in child abuse and neglect cases:

1. determining the history of abuse or neglect
2. assessing the resulting harm to the child
3. assessing a parent's current capacity to provide for a child
4. predicting future risk and treatment response for children and parents.

In discussing the harm that may have occurred to the child as a result of abuse or neglect, the author indicates that the questions require "some specific areas of expertise as well as careful attention to problems of developmental psychopathology and comorbidity." He notes the expert must answer two questions:

First, a careful diagnostic assessment with special attention to the identification both of specific disorders and of general characteristics of the child's psychological functioning, and second, the articulation of the specific likely origins of disorder and deficit in the individual child, taking account both of the apparent history of abuse or neglect and of other elements of the child's development that may have been less than ideal[14].

The author gives suggestions on how to conduct the examination and assessment as well as in structuring the forensic evaluation reports. However, he does not go into the means by which further harm can be minimized or avoided during this assessment procedure.

7.6   Juvenile Offenders

The examination of juvenile defenders is complicated by the fact that the laws have changed regarding certification to adult court or decertification to juvenile court. Issues abound with respect to the evaluation of juveniles charged with crime and the death penalty. Changes also have occurred regarding whether juveniles can receive the death penalty. Ethical concerns on the part of forensic psychiatrists have deterred a number of forensic psychiatrists from becoming involved in capital cases involving juveniles. Finally, issues of treatment of juveniles in the correctional system reflect concerns about harming juveniles within the system.

DePrato and Hammer discuss the role of the assessor in conducting the examination and assessment of juvenile offenders:

> The results of the clinician's evaluation and treatment recommendations have serious implications for the child's life. An adequate evaluation will direct treatment to reduce risk factors while enhancing protective factors, thus minimizing the possibility of the youth's further involvement in delinquent activities. Inadequate evaluation and treatment will have little impact upon the juvenile's situation and often leads to treatment failure, resulting in serious legal consequences for the youth, such as incarceration [15].

7.7   Decertification

In criminal cases, one may have a problem with children if one is examining for the prosecution to see whether there should be a waiver from adult court to juvenile court or vice versa. The prosecution is interested in protecting the community, and by doing so, puts the juvenile in an adult situation where he/she would have a longer sentence.

On one day, I was asked to examine two separate youngsters. In one case, I was requested by the defense attorney to see his client, a 14-year-old boy who had killed his mother. He had come home from school at lunchtime, taken his father's shotgun, loaded it, waited for his mother to come home, confronted her, and told her that he was upset with the way she was treating him, showing preference for his 12-year-old sister. He said he did not like it, he was tired of it, and he was going to do something about it. At that point, she had taunted him, telling him he was no good and what was he doing with a gun, and that if he really felt the way he said, that he should go ahead and shoot, which he did, killing her. Even though he was only 14 and he was angry with his mother, he was not psychotic or mentally disturbed, except that he acted out his passion and his conflict against his mother. I could not recommend that he remain in juvenile court.

In the other case, I was asked by the prosecution to examine a 16-year-old boy who had shot his father in a department store in a large shopping mall. The family had gone out to celebrate the youngster's sixteenth birthday. On the way home, he asked if he could have a music tape recording that he wanted for his birthday. His father, who had taunted, him, teased him, and threatened him with a loaded gun on several occasions, had denied him his request and began berating him verbally in front of others in this crowded shopping area. The boy was in tears, ran back to the car, which was not locked, found the loaded weapon under the passenger seat where father had regularly kept it. He came back into the department store, confronted his father with the loaded gun in front of a number of people who scattered, but witnessed his shooting his father.

He aimed the gun at his father and was in tears when his father told him that he was no good and that he would never shoot because he did not have the guts. The boy was angry, but also quite disturbed, having been threatened with his life by his father on several occasions with the same gun he now pointed at his father. He shot his father once, dropped the gun in shock, ran to his father's falling body, hugged his father, kissing him, telling his father that that was something he could never do while his father was alive. It was clear to me that this was a boy who had been traumatized by a sadistic father, one who not only threatened him, but also his mother and younger sister. He confessed that he felt only relief after his father was gone, because he no longer had to fear his father's threats and worry about father killing him and the rest of the family. On the other hand, he was also quite disturbed at his loss of control and was highly amenable to treatment and rehabilitation.

On one day, I had examined two youngsters, both of whom had killed parents. One for the defense where I felt I could not recommend he stay in juvenile court, and the other for the prosecution in which I felt remaining in juvenile court was necessary to help the youngster.

In the first case, the 14-year-old boy was waived to adult court, stood trial as an adult, and was found guilty of killing his mother. However, under the law, he could spend only until the age of 21 in prison for his punishment for murder. On the other hand, the 16-year-old who remained in juvenile court, was given a two-year suspended sentence for killing his father and mandated to treatment until the treatment was completed by the time he was 21 years of age. Both individuals had limited sentences, one for therapy and the other for punishment. These are two examples of how a forensic psychiatrist may evaluate juveniles charged with crimes and either be helpful or at least minimize the harm done when therapy is not available.

Ratner [16] refers to the United States Supreme Court case of *Roper v. Simmons* [17] in 2005 that does not allow the execution of minors under the age of 18. Prior to that case, he notes, 19 states had laws allowing the execution of minors of 16 years or older. He states that one had to be waived or transferred to adult court in order to be eligible for the death penalty in those states. However, he also noted it was getting "systematically easier for a juvenile to end up there." He concludes that *Roper* took the death penalty off the table for all who committed a crime prior to their eighteenth birthday. He states that while juvenile offenders may still get transferred to adult court, they cannot be put to death. He states this has "proven a great relief to psychiatrists who are ethically opposed to the death penalty in general and for minors in particular. Those who participate in transfer hearings had great difficulty doing so with the realization that transfer to adult court could be tantamount to a death sentence. Those working for the government, and expected to recommend transfer when warranted, were in an impossible position, knowing that their recommendation could lead to death" [16].

Defense-appointed psychiatrists could be upset if their efforts failed to retain a juvenile who was later condemned to death, or caused them to "withdraw their appearances if their evaluation led them to find little chance for rehabilitation" [15].

In a recent study, Washburn *et al.* [18] showed that youths processed in juvenile court had fewer psychiatric disorders than those processed in adult criminal court. The participants were between 13 and 18 years of age and involved 1440 youths processed in juvenile court, and 275 in adult criminal court. The results show that males, African Americans, Hispanics, and older youths had greater odds of being processed in adult criminal court than females, non-Hispanic whites, and younger youths, even after the analyses controlled for felony level violent crime. The authors found that among youths processed in adult criminal court, 68% had at least one psychiatric disorder, and 43% had two or more types of disorders. Among youths processed in adult criminal court, those sentenced to prison had significantly greater odds than those receiving a less severe sentence of having a disruptive behavior disorder, a substance use disorder, or comorbid affective and anxiety disorders.

The authors concluded that "community and correctional systems must be prepared to provide psychiatric services to youths transferred to adult criminal court, and especially youths sentenced to prison" [18]. The authors also stress that when developing and implementing services, the providers must consider the "disproportionate representation of individuals from racial-ethnic-minority groups in the transfer process."

7.8 Sexual Abuse of Children

Children who are sexually abused require especially sensitive, careful ethical assessment within a larger context of:

1. the legal situation;
2. family psychodynamics;
3. age of the victim;
4. the manner in which the assessment is conducted, including collateral interviews, review of records, and numbers of times the victim is interviewed or examined, either alone or in conjunction with others;
5. the identity of the alleged perpetrator(s).

These are especially important cases, because the system may tend, in some jurisdictions, to doubly harm the victim by adhering to various principles that protect the rights of the alleged perpetrators, sometimes demanding the victim face his or her perpetrator in court.

In 1988, the Supreme Court held that a defendant's Sixth Amendment Right to confront his accuser precluded screening the child witness from the defendant without a special showing of need (*Coy v. Iowa*, 1988) [19]. Two years later, in 1990, the Court found that the trauma to the child of testifying could override the defendant's right of face-to-face confrontation in particular cases and upheld the statute, allowing allegedly abused children to testify in a separate room and have their testimony televised to the judge, jury, defendant, and spectators (*Maryland v. Craig*, 1990) [20]. In that case, the court noted, "Trauma to the witness as proved by expert opinion was given sufficient weight to overcome the defendant's right to a face-to-face confrontation" [20].

Subsequent cases focused on the protection of the child in such cases. They include *Idaho v. Wright* (1990) [21] and *White v. Illinois* (1992) [22] in which the court allowed others to testify about what the child had said regarding her abuse as a "spontaneous utterance" exception to the general bar against hearsay evidence. The child's statements then were introduced without her having to testify in court, thus minimizing harm to the child.

Thus, the courts have generally tried to balance the right of someone facing his or her accuser with the rights of children. In that regard, some courts have allowed closed circuit TV or videotape in order to protect the child and not have him or her confront their accuser.

A study in Iowa, utilizing a questionnaire that was sent to the presidents of all area child abuse and neglect councils as well as other personnel working with sexually abused children, revealed that "approximately 21% of the victims perceived the questioning and investigation as being harmful, while approximately 53% saw it as helpful. The ratings of helpfulness were not correlated with the age of the victim, the presence of a supportive adult during questioning, the number of abuse incidents, whether or not the interviews were videotaped, and whether or not the perpetrator was a family member. Testifying in court and high numbers of interviews were associated with more negative ratings" [23].

In responding to the question of harm by testifying, Tedesco and Schnell [24] state, "The experience could be cathartic, provide a feeling of control, provide an indication and symbolically put an end to an unpleasant experience." In essence, they feel that testifying may have a positive effect on the child that ultimately outweighs negative aspects.

These authors give examples that childhood victimization "is a lifelong struggle" whether or not the child testifies against the perpetrator. They note, in their experience, cases in which children had testified with positive results. As an example, they cite, "the three year old who witnessed her mother's murder and continued, six years later, to lament that she was unable 'to help mommie,' but takes pride in being able to tell what happened to the judge" [24].

The same article cites traditional attempts to minimize stress on the child who testifies:

> More recently, the judicial system has demonstrated an awareness of the literature that has identified the arguments against childhood testimony. Courts have attempted to minimize the stress by providing child advocates, courtroom visits by the child, screening techniques, closed circuit testimony, role playing, and the courtroom presence of supportive adults. These have all been initiated to reduce a child's stress and are welcome evidence of an increased sensitivity to the needs of children [25].

An article in *Pediatrics* (1992) [26], is a guide as to how to treat the child in the legal system:

> Children may be confused by negatively worded statements. They may also be eager to please, anxious to provide the 'right' answer and may have a tendency to choose either the first or the last option when given a number from which to select. Therefore, it is essential that clearly worded questions that encourage children to provide answers that will be viewed non-judgmentally are used. Correct answers or a scenario should not be suggested as children may be influenced and are prone to suggestibility [27].

In a very comprehensive article, Shapiro makes recommendations for interviewing sexually abused children. Clinically practical questions are phrased so that children can understand and answer them, and suggestions are made for introducing and concluding the interview. However, the recommendations are more for "obtaining information in a sensitive manner, but not so much for preventing further harm." The author states, "In general, diagnostic interviews are stressful procedures which are performed for the sake of the future goal of facilitating case management and intervention; nonetheless, these interviews can also be reassuring and helpful for the abused child" [28].

Weissman instructs us how to conduct a sensitive examination "protecting the rights of the accused as well as not harming the child" [29]. In this paper, the author refers to a secondary trauma and proposed hearsay exceptions, "on the assumption the child victim-witnesses are traumatized by testifying in court, especially in the presence of the accused, hearsay exceptions and the use of protective measures have been proposed in several jurisdictions. Psychological research has studied the capabilities of children to testify on the emotional effects of their involvement in the legal process." Methods of conducting appropriate examinations in such cases are discussed. The author concludes, "The mental health professional has the opportunity to benefit the fact finder by providing comprehensive, technically neutral, independent examinations in cases where child sexual abuse is charged ... Critical issues pertaining to the interests of vulnerable children and the rights of the accused are at stake. Both demand the highest respect and protection" [29].

Jenkins and Howell have reviewed the literature regarding child sexual abuse examinations, and they propose a more objective and stringent standard of care:

> *Current limitations in sexual abuse examinations include examiner bias, faulty procedures or diagnostic materials, and varied or conflicting roles of the judicial, social service, and mental health systems. Examiners in such cases should have adequate and specific training, be a neutral party appointed by the court, record the proceedings, and have access not only to the alleged victim, but also to the accused and to other parties during the examination [30].*

The authors recommend how to conduct the examination of the child without leading the child and without suggesting things to the child, and also how to interview others, but they do not indicate specifically how to minimize harm. They are more concerned about the sources of error that might occur due to "the highly sensitive and emotional nature of the allegations. Examiners should use caution to be sure that bias and suggestibility are minimized at every phase of the evaluation, maintaining the stance of neutrality and healthy skepticism until all of the data are in" [30]. They point to the essential differences between the child therapist and the forensic examiner:

> *The position of the examiner is not to be a therapist or child advocate, but one to arrive at objective conclusions based on unbiased data. As sexual abuse examinations become more objective and less biased or emotionally charged, the system for dealing with such allegations will function more cleanly and will better serve the purpose for which it was intended [30].*

Burton and Myers [31] point to the following controversial areas in child sexual abuse cases:

- psychic damages
- false allegations
- improper investigatory techniques
- use of anatomical dolls
- admissibility of expert testimony
  - — hearsay testimony
  - — competency of minors to testify.

In discussing the psychic trauma that occurs following sexual abuse, the authors cite Summit [32] and his "Child Sexual Abuse Accommodation Syndrome," in which he identified five progressive stages:

- secrecy
- helplessness
- entrapment and accommodation
- delayed, conflicted, unconvincing disclosure
- retraction.

There is much controversy about the issue of children who have complained of being sexually abused facing their alleged perpetrators in court. Studies have been conducted to determine the effect of such confrontation on the victims of sexual abuse. In a 1997 review article, the authors studied the effects of interviewing children in the setting of sexual abuse allegations: "In a number of highly publicized sexual abuse cases, when juries have found guilt, Appellate Courts have reversed convictions" [33]. They cite the case of *State v. Michaels* [34], in which the New Jersey Supreme Court, in 1994, found several instances of suggestive and coercive interviewing and declared the children's testimony must meet the same test the court had set previously for hypnotically refreshed testimony: "Once a criminal defendant raises the likelihood of inappropriate questioning of a child, the state has to prove by clear and convincing evidence that the testimony is valid before it can be admitted."

In discussing the issue of whether children should testify directly facing their perpetrators of sexual abuse, the authors note, "The children's greatest fear about testifying involved facing the defendant." The study they conducted showed that a seven month follow-up of children who testified "evidenced greater disturbance than children who did not testify, and lack of improvement was associated with testifying multiple times, less maternal support, and less collaborating evidence. Counseling the children did not improve their condition" [33].

What this means is that we can harm children by having them testify directly facing the defendant rather than protecting them by other means the courts have devised.

Renshaw [35] has developed a child sex history document consisting of two pages that is quite detailed and used as a supplement to routine medical psychosocial histories. She also addresses the ethical issues involved in such cases. She notes, "Some pitfalls in history taking are to be remembered by all who work in this difficult and highly emotional arena of child sexual abuse. Children try to please adults as part of their normal security-seeking behavior; therefore, it can be easy to mislead a child." Next, she notes the inner world of a child is different from that of the adult. "For a child, symbolism, fantasy, fusion and confusion, make believe, and primitive thinking are pathways as they learn to incorporate daily experiences and information to make sense of the world around them." Her concern is that in our culture we have stimulated the "good touch bad touch" phenomenon such that some good touches are avoided for fear of being accused of "bad touching." She believes some of this may be harmful to children.

Appelbaum [36] hails the opinion of Justice Sandra Day O'Connor in *Coy v. Iowa* and her indication that the rights of the children need to be protected even while protecting the rights of the defendant. Appelbaum cautions forensic experts working in this field not to make predictions that they may not be able to support with scientific evidence. He states, "Many clinicians hold strong views about the impact of courtroom testimony on child victims, but almost no empirical data are available to back up their beliefs. No published follow-up studies have examined the impact of testimony on child victims of abuse" [36].

Yates [37] declares, "Children may be helped or harmed by testifying. The risk of further traumatization can be minimized through the judge's use of discretionary power, inclusion of professionals trained in child development in the investigative and court process, and use of videotaping or one way screens." The author notes, "The trauma for the young child witness can be lessened in spite of the legal system's disinclination to change. Following Colorado's lead, several states now allow children to be examined in a separate chamber with the judge and opposing counsel while the accused views the proceedings on a video monitor or through a one way screen."

The author raises the constitutional question of the defendant's rights to consult his attorney and to confront his accuser "may be violated by placing the child and the defense attorney in a separate chamber ... The vast majority of jurisdictions continue to demand the face to face confrontation as specified in the Constitution. Some jurisdictions require videotaped depositions of children in sexual assault cases, which ... may eliminate the need for the child to appear in court" [37].

The author recommends the use of a person trained in child development to conduct the initial examination which would be taped and used in place of the child's testimony should the case go to court.

Yates refers to the case of the three-year-old girl in Colorado who was molested and abandoned in a cesspit and the treating psychiatrist serving as the court examiner questioned the child from behind a one-way mirror while responding to the attorney's questions through a tiny transmitter in his ear. She notes that this was a remarkable feat, the constitutionality of which "must be tested at the Appellate Court level. However, if child witnesses are to be humanely treated and protected from further damage, further involvement of child psychiatrists is clearly indicated" [38].

As a general ethical guideline Quinn [39] indicates,

> *The primary goal of investigatory interviewing is to document the chronology, psychosocial context and consistency of an allegation ... The investigator must maintain internal independence by being open, honest, and unbiased in gathering data and hearing the child's account of his or her experience. Interviewers should utilize the same principles as scientific investigators by ruling in or out alternate hypotheses as well as acknowledging the limitations of their data [39].*

Quinn further states, "Interviewers must be careful to avoid role confusions. The interviewer must remember that he or she is a forensic examiner, not a therapist or child advocate for any particular case." In summary, she states, "Clinicians receiving referral of a case involving an allegation of child sexual abuse must define their role for themselves and all participants." Further, she states, the clinician "must bring a developmental perspective to interview a child about allegations of abuse. There are well documented age related differences in memory, suggestibility, reasoning, knowledge, range of experience, and emotional maturity." She concludes, "Conducting such assessments in child sexual abuse can be harmful to the child, depending on how the interview is conducted, how the interview is done, and whether the child recants at a later interview or whether the accusation is 'improbable' with the facts noted" [39].

In summary, these articles in the literature focus on how to interview, how to minimize harm to the child who must be a witness for a number of reasons. One is clearly to not traumatize the child any more than necessary; two, to try to get as much truthfulness as possible; and three, not to have suggested to the child various issues that may not be truthful.

Thus, there are two issues here: One is the manner in which the interview takes place and how the psychiatrist handles child cases and, secondly, more importantly, the impact on the child for even being in court. Children's presence in court, of course, is not of their own doing, but the doing of others, either those who abused them, harmed them, injured them, or because their parents are going through a divorce.

In conducting assessments of victims of childhood sexual abuse, it is important not to lead the child to give the answers desired by the interviewer. Harm can come to the child victim if the interview is not done properly, such that it would not be admissible in court or would be unbelievable if presented to the jury.

7.8.1 Case Examples

There is a case of a sergeant in the United States Army who had been invited to stay at a friend's home at another Army base. His friend, also a sergeant, had three daughters, all of whom lived at home. The sergeant had a great deal to drink with his friend during and after dinner. He slept over that night, and during the middle of the night, he had to get up to go to the bathroom. Inadvertently, he went into the wrong room, walking into one daughter's room. She later alleged that he had touched her sexually while he was in her room. He had no memory of the encounter and no memory of walking into the wrong room. He was arrested for indecent assault, endangering a minor and other related charges. Because it happened on an Army base and he was on active duty, he faced a court martial. The evidence against him was exclusively the statement made by the six-year-old daughter, who claimed that she was inappropriately touched by him that night.

The daughter's statement was taken by a young social worker who had been employed for less than a year by the Prosecutor's Office. She had no experience in interviewing a child sexual abuse victim. It was clear from reviewing the tape that the interview of the child was not professional in that she led the child and suggested things to her to make the statement absolutely meaningless. During the course of the court martial, the videotape was shown to the members of the court martial board and stopped every few minutes to reveal where the leading questions were given and the answers responded and conformed clearly to the questions asked. Because of the leading nature of the questions given to the child, the Board found the statement incredible and, therefore, found the sergeant not guilty of the crimes charged. It was never known whether the child was, in fact, sexually abused or not, because the statement was not trusted by the court martial board. Thus, harm was done to the child by the interviewer, who did not know how to properly interview a child sexual victim without leading her to get the answers that she wanted. One must be extremely careful in conducting such examinations in order to avoid leading the child in such a manner that her statement would not be acceptable.

Another case involves the examination of an eight-year-old girl who was mentally retarded and had not seen her biological mother for some time. She had been living with a foster family, and DHS[4] wanted to terminate her mother's parental rights and give the child up for adoption to the foster family. The forensic child psychologist was asked to do an examination regarding bonding of the child; it was a very sensitive exam, and the judge was concerned about harm coming to the child, so he put some limitations and restrictions on the examination. He indicated that the child was to be seen only for a short period of time, the mother was not to be present unless changes were made, and the psychologist had to see the mother with the child in order to assess the bonding issue.

The child had not seen the mother for some time, and there was some question about the father having sexually abused the child. The father was seen by another forensic psychologist who indicated, after psychological testing and examination, that in his opinion the father had not sexually abused his daughter. She had claimed that it happened and said it was both anal and vaginal, and an examination by a pediatrician showed that she had some tearing of the hymen to corroborate the vaginal, but nothing to show there was any damage in the anal area. She did seem unhappy with the father. The makeup of the family was this: Father was married to another woman and had children with that woman. He then had an affair with the girl's mother, who became pregnant and the girl was born. She was raised by the mother for the first few years, but then she became a problem, became depressed and had difficulty, so father said he had to leave his wife and family and move in with girlfriend and daughter in order to help raise their daughter. It was around that time that the child was seen to be doing poorly in school, her IQ measure dropped about 20 points, and the parents worried that something had happened to her.

DHS got involved, and the allegation of sexual abuse arose. Father was investigated, but no criminal charges were brought. DHS said that mother had to get father out of the house and she had to go for sex therapy. Mother would never admit that she knew that father did anything to their daughter, and if she did not admit that, she could not stay in therapy. Without the therapy, she would not get her daughter back. So there was an effort to keep the daughter with the foster family and away from the mother, but the court wanted to know, at the request of the family, the bonding of mother and daughter. The psychologist found that the daughter bonded very well with the foster family and later found that the daughter, in a very sensitive way, was able to bond with mother. The psychologist had instructed the child that she did not have to see mother, but if she would, the psychologist would be there and would protect her, and so on. The mother was

---

[4] United States Department of Human Services.

very sensitive about not pushing too hard, and handled it well. The child kept moving closer to the mother, showing her mother her scrap book and her picture book. Mother then was allowed to take a picture of the daughter, which she had not done for over five years. Two things happened here: the child psychologist's professionalism allowed the examination to proceed in a manner that was sensitive and not too harmful to the child. However, if the intent of DHS was to terminate parental rights and to give the child to the foster family for adoption, then introducing her after several years to her mother, whom she knew about, could only work in the opposite direction and be confusing to her.

This was the case that stimulated my interest in writing about minimizing harm during the forensic psychiatric examination. I felt the sensitivity of the forensic child psychologist presenting this case was such that she could minimize the harm to the child while making the effort to reunite this family. She recognized there would be some strain and some difficulty after many years of separation, but handled the case with such care and sensitivity as to minimize any harm to the child during the reintroduction phase to her mother. The long-term gain, of course, was important inasmuch as the child and mother were reunited in a successful manner.

7.9   Bias in the Examination of Children

Horner and others [40] present a case of child forensic psychiatrists evaluating "the likelihood of a three-year-old child having been sexually molested by her father, as alleged by her mother, when she was two years old." All of the experts claimed to have qualifications and experiences in the field of diagnosing and treating child sexual abuse victims. The clinical case was presented in two different ways: one, a detailed presentation by the child psychiatrist who evaluated the youngster, and another where the case was presented to child psychiatric experts. When the survey of the responders was taken, the authors found an extreme range of estimated likelihood of molestation by the experts who responded. "The experts then gave recommendations to the court how the court should regulate further child-father contact, and they were similarly varied" [40]. The authors note the study reveals the biases that exist among examiners regarding sexual abuse. The authors also note that of all the studies they have conducted in this area, this is the only one to adduce possible evidence of gender-related opinion-formation. It should be noted that one of the female respondents recommended custody of the child be shifted to the father.

The importance of this study is that there is bias in the evaluation process and that the experts do not always get it right. The recommendations made to the court vary also, and may depend upon the bias and background of the experts. Thus, the child may be harmed if the expert gets it wrong because of his or her own inherent bias.

7.10   Specific Concerns about Child Forensic Psychiatric Examinations

I have been very concerned about professional abuse in these cases in which the professional mental health expert, guided by his or her skills, background and experience, proclaims that he or she "knows" what has happened when, in fact, there are so many variables that it may be impossible to determine whether a child was, in fact, sexually abused by a particular person. In one case, a father was so accused and was clearly not involved sexually with his daughter, but was kept from her for several years. It was clear from the videotapes of the visitation with the father that the child was not afraid of him and was not "disgusted" by his presence, did not recoil when he came into the room, and she showed a warmth and love that would not be present if she had been sexually abused as claimed. When the child was returned to visitation with the father, it was even more striking, because she continued to show love for him, was warm and friendly with him during reunification and for several years following. However, it is clear that she, as well as he, was hurt by the intervention by the court to "protect" the child because of the accusations that were clearly unfounded.

Another case example involves an eight-year-old girl who was the victim in the custody dispute between her mother and father. The parents were not married, both professional, both very bright, and both very caring. However, the mother had considerable concern about the father, whom she accused of sexually molesting their daughter when the daughter was between two and three years of age. The child and the father were evaluated and the judge found, as did the Children and Youth Association, that the accusations were not founded, and no action was taken. The mother had hired several child forensic psychiatrists and psychologists, all of whom gave reports that there was indeed sexual abuse even though the father was never evaluated and the child was not seen by some of the experts. There was also an accusation of parental alienation syndrome by the mother against the father.

One forensic psychologist did examine the child a day before a visit with the father and the day following that visit. The psychologist's report noted that the child was appropriate, well mannered, and without difficulty communicating the day before the visit, but found that the day after visitation with the father, the child was "psychotic, incoherent, and extremely upset." There were some allegations about sexual contact as well in the communications. Other experts were then consulted to examine the child and the accusations against father continued even though the Children and Youth authority found no evidence for sexual abuse. Finally, the judge heard all the evidence, dismissed the case for lack of evidence of child sexual abuse.

This case is presented primarily to show that children can be harmed when there is such animosity between the parents or when one parent charges the other with sexual abuse. It is confusing to the child when she is told that some experts have found that she was abused and others found that she was not, and the judge determined that she was not abused. In addition, examination of the father showed no evidence for pedophilic interest or behavior, either prior to or since the accusation. The father was given custody of the child, and no further difficulties or charges against the father were made. Court appointed experts noted a good relationship between the child and her father as well as between the child and her mother.

From what sources do these accusations stem and how do experts evaluate the accuracy, the veracity and factual nature of such accusations? There are psychological tests for sexual perversions or sexually violent predators that are administered by psychologists who can give reasonable predictions about a person's sexual orientation, sexual proclivity, and sexual difficulties. However, the testing cannot tell whether or not abuse has occurred. The question arises then: How do we utilize our skills, our professional experience and the tools we have available in order to effect a just conclusion or opinion in such a case where accusations are made and variable results occur?

Thus, it is my plea to my colleagues to be very cautious in these most difficult cases that can appear to be obvious, and one may feel that he or she is serving a just purpose by pointing the finger at the accused and protecting or rescuing the child from the predator or the sexual perpetrator. In fact, however, when no such abuse has occurred, the rescue becomes a fantasy that leads to separation of the child from a loving parent. This is not, in my opinion, in the best interest of the child, is an abuse of professional power and is harmful to the child involved.

Therefore, it behooves the forensic child psychiatric examiner in sexual abuse cases to make every effort to minimize further harm to the child who is already traumatized by the sexual abuse and by some of the procedures within the criminal justice system. By adhering to the ethical guidelines of the various organizations noted, including the AMA, the APA, AAPL, AACAP, we can minimize the harm to child and adolescent victims of sexual abuse.

7.11 Summary

In summary, there are a number of instances in which child forensic psychiatrists and psychologists become involved in cases involving children and adolescents. We have skills, experience, and professional tools at our disposal to help the courts in making a just decision. However, we also have the power to harm the child or adolescent if our skills are misused, abused, or we are not thorough in our assessments. One manner in which we can adhere to the concept of minimizing harm to children and adolescents, a very vulnerable population, is to cling to the ethical guidelines of the American Academy of Psychiatry and the Law. We must maintain or strive for neutrality and objectivity, honesty, lack of bias whenever possible, openness and thoroughness in our evaluations and assessments. We should be open to the fact that we may be wrong, and be flexible in reviewing newer evidence that might shed light on the situation, causing us to amend our conclusions.

References

1. Tedesco, J.F. and Schnell, S.V. (1987) Children's reactions to sex abuse investigation and litigation. *Child Abuse and Neglect*, **11**, 267–72.
2. Haller, L.H. (2002). The Forensic Evaluation and Court Testimony. *Child and Adolescent Psychiatric* Clinics, **11**, 689–704.
3. See Ref. [2], p. 689.
4. Ratner, R.A. (2005) Ethical issues in forensic psychiatry with children and adolescents. *Psychiatric Times*, **23**(14), 3–5, at p. 3.
5. Enzer, N. (1985) Ethics in child psychiatry: An overview, in *Emerging Issues in Child Psychiatry and the Law* (eds. D.H. Schetky and E.P. Benedek), Brunner/Mazel, New York, pp. 3–21.
6. See Ref. [4], p. 5.
7. Goldzband, M.G. (1982) *Consulting in Child Custody: An Introduction to the Ugliest Litigation for Mental Health Professionals*, Lexington Books, D.C. Heath and Company, Lexington.
8. Gardner, R.A. (1998) *Parental Alienation Syndrome*, Creative Therapeutics, Inc., Cresskill.
9. *Palmor v. Sidoti*, 466 US 429, (1984).
10. Miller, G.H. (2002) The psychological best interest of the child is not the legal best interest. *Journal of the American Academy of Psychiatry and the Law*, **30**, 196–200.
11. See Ref. [10], p. 200.
12. See Ref. [10], p. 196.
13. Barnum, R. (1997) A suggested framework for forensic consultation in cases of child abuse and neglect. *Journal of the American Academy of Psychiatry and the Law*, **25**, 581–93.
14. See Ref. [13], p. 586.
15. DePrato, D.K. and Hammer, J.H. (2002) Assessment and treatment of juvenile offenders, in *Principles and Practice of Child and Adolescent Forensic Psychiatry* (eds. D.H. Schetky and E.P. Benedek), American Psychiatric Publishing, Inc., Washington, DC, pp. 267–78.
16. Ratner, R. (2005) Ethical issues in forensic psychiatry with children and adolescents. *Psychiatric Times*, 5.
17. *Roper v. Simmons*, 112 SW 3d 397, (2005).
18. Washburn, J.J., Teplin, L.A., Voss, L.S. *et al.* (2008) Psychiatric disorders among detained youths: A comparison of youths processed in Juvenile Court and Adult Criminal Court. *Psychiatric Services*, **59**, 965–73.
19. *Coy v. Iowa*, 487 US 1012, 108 S. Ct. 2798, (1988).
20. *Maryland v. Craig*, 497 US 836, 110 S. Ct. 3157, (1990).
21. *Idaho v. Wright*, 497 US 805, (1990).
22. *White v. Illinois*, 502 US 346, (1992).
23. Tedesco, J.F. and Schnell, S.V. (1987) Children's reactions to sex abuse investigation and litigation. *Child Abuse and Neglect*, **11**, 267–72.
24. See Ref. [23], p. 270.
25. See Ref. [23], p. 271.
26. American Academy of Pediatrics Committee on Psychosocial Aspects of Child and Family Health (1992) The child as a witness. *Pediatrics*, **89**, 513–15.
27. See Ref. [26], p. 514.

28. Shapiro, J.P. (1991) Interviewing children about psychological issues associated with sexual abuse. *Psychotherapy*, **28**, 55–66.
29. Weissman, H.N. (1991) Forensic psychological examination of the child witness in cases of alleged sexual abuse. *American Journal of Orthopsychiatry*, **61**(1), 48–58.
30. Jenkins, P.H. and Howell, R.J. (1994) Child sexual abuse examinations: proposed guidelines for a standard of care. *Bulletin of the American Academy of Psychiatry and the Law*, **22**, 5–17.
31. Burton, K. and Myers, W.C. (1992) Child sexual abuse and forensic psychiatry: evolving and controversial issues. *Bulletin of the American Academy of Psychiatry and the Law*, **20**, 439–53.
32. Summit, R. (1983) The child sexual abuse accommodation syndrome. *Child Abuse and Neglect*, **7**, 177–92.
33. AACAP Official Action (1997) Practice parameters for the forensic evaluation of children and adolescents who may have been physically or sexually abused. *Journal of the American Academy of Child and Adolescent Psychiatry*, **36**, (Suppl. 10), 37S–56S.
34. *State v. Michaels*, 136 NJ 299, (1994).
35. Renshaw, D.C. (1987) Evaluating suspected cases of child sexual abuse. *Psychiatric Annals*, **17**, 262–70.
36. Appelbaum, P.S. (1989) Protecting child witnesses in sexual abuse cases. *Hospital and Community Psychiatry*, **40**, 13–14.
37. Yates, A. (1987) Should young children testify in cases of sexual Abuse? *The American Journal of Psychiatry*, **144**(4), 476–80.
38. See Ref. [37], p. 478.
39. Quinn, K. (2002) Interviewing children for suspected sexual abuse, in *Principles and Practice of Child and Adolescent Forensic Psychiatry* (eds. D. Schetky and E. Benedek), The American Psychiatric Press, Washington, DC, p. 152.
40. Horner, T.M., Guyer, M.J., and Kelter, N.M. (1993) The biases of child sexual abuse experts: believing is seeing. *Bulletin of the American Academy of Psychiatry and the Law*, **21**, 281–92.

8 The Elderly, the Mentally Retarded, and the Severely Mentally Disabled

Robert L. Sadoff

University of Pennsylvania School of Medicine, Philadelphia, USA

8.1 Introduction

In a prior chapter we discussed children and adolescents who are often involved in the judicial system because of the behaviors of others, especially their parents, or sometimes because of their own behavior leading to criminal charges. We have seen what can happen to children and adolescents when the psychiatric examiner is not sensitive to the plight of the child in a domestic relations conflict or when the child is charged as an adult in criminal court.

There are other populations that are equally vulnerable within the judicial system. Perhaps the most obvious are the elderly, who may be abused by family members and others who are able to take advantage of those with dementia and those of advanced age who have physical disabilities. The elderly also form a vulnerable population when examined by forensic experts. The plea here is to minimize the harm to the elderly who are involved either in civil or criminal matters.

Other vulnerable populations include the mentally retarded, who may not clearly understand the significance of their involvement in the criminal justice system when they are charged with various crimes or are victims of criminal behavior. Clearly, the mentally ill defendant or plaintiff may also be at a disadvantage within the system, unless treated with sensitivity and respect. As in the concepts of racism and sexism, Birnbaum [1] has coined the phrase "sanism," in which he refers to

Ethical Issues in Forensic Psychiatry: Minimizing Harm by Robert L. Sadoff
© 2011 John Wiley & Sons, Ltd

the bias people have against the mentally ill. He also is considered the "father of mental health law," inasmuch as he initiated the drive for rights of the mentally ill within the legal system. His pioneering efforts have led to radical changes in mental health law that have benefitted the mentally ill who are involved in the legal system.

This treatise is not about mental health law, as there are various publications that address those issues quite well [2]. This is about the vulnerability of the mentally ill and the mentally retarded and others within the criminal and civil justice system who require special management.

8.2   The Elderly

We have seen a number of cases of elder abuse in which the victim has been traumatized, neglected, or even sexually and physically abused by caretakers and/or other family members. It is often difficult to obtain necessary information from such victims, who may have had serious dementia or other mental and emotional problems prior to the discovery of their victimization. How does one interview and assess the damages to an elderly person with Alzheimer's or other forms of dementia? Are there valid psychological tests that can be utilized to assess the mental state of such individuals? What other collateral interviews are necessary in order to arrive at a valid forensic psychiatric assessment?

Sometimes, the elderly are killed. The perpetrator may also be an elderly individual who requires sensitive examination. We have seen cases in which elderly parents are killed by their adult children because the parent has become a burden to the caretaker. Often, these adult children are in their seventies and the parents were well into their nineties. Sometimes, the perpetrator is the spouse of the elderly, who cannot tolerate watching his wife suffer from the ravages of cancer or the wife cannot tolerate the care and suffering of her demented husband.

In addition, elderly persons can be victimized by others who intend to unduly influence them, to steal from them, or to take advantage of them. In will contests, elderly persons with weakened intellect have been known to be unduly influenced by persons who have an intimate relationship with them and influence them to change their will. One may not be able to examine the elderly in such cases, because the will would not come to light until after the person's demise. How does the forensic examiner assess weakened intellect in such an elderly individual after death? One needs to use collateral information, the observations of others, and whatever audio or videotapes are available to shed light on the mental state of the testator. Sometimes, the issue is not weakened intellect with respect to undue influence, but the competency of the elderly person to write the will or to understand the provisions of the will written by his or her attorney.

Elderly persons are also taken advantage of by unscrupulous retailers and others who steal from them and attempt to take their property or their money. Elderly people occasionally will sign away property without competency to do so, or they may buy things they do not need, because they are of weakened intellect and are unduly influenced by others.

Elderly individuals may require assessment for competency to enter into a contract, to write a will or to manage their own affairs. The assessment of the elderly should be conducted on more than one occasion and at different times of the day, whenever possible. It is well known that the elderly may be more alert in the morning and, therefore, more "competent." The old person who has some difficulty with memory may not be competent at the end of the day when fatigued.

As noted, the elderly may be involved in criminal matters as well. They may be charged with killing parents or spouses for altruistic reasons. Euthanasia committed by the elderly should not be confused with insanity. One has to ask the question whether the elderly individual knew what he or she was doing and knew that it was wrong when they killed their spouse. The defendant may have a strong belief that what they were doing was the right thing for their parents or their spouse in order to "put them out of their misery." This is especially true if the spouse is demented with Alzheimer's or is suffering from the ravages of cancer or other debilitating, painful chronic diseases.

In conducting the assessment of such individuals, the evaluator should ask specifically if the perpetrator had delusions or a serious mental illness that led to the violent, destructive behavior rather than just a belief that the parent or spouse would be better off without the suffering. Some people cherish life even with pain, and should not be euthanized because it will be easier and more convenient for the survivor. Sometimes there is an agreement that the one who does the killing will then kill themselves in a murder-suicide pact with the spouse. Often, the suicide is not successful and the survivor is then charged with the killing of their spouse.

8.2.1   Case Examples

In one recent case, an elderly man had been charged in the death of his wife, having shot her in the head one time to "put her out of her misery." The psychiatrist evaluating him for the defense concluded that he had a cognitive disorder as well as depression and PTSD from caring for her. PTSD is the result of a serious life threatening trauma that affects a person with identifiable characteristics and symptoms. This particular man did not have symptoms of PTSD, though he had been stressed (perhaps not traumatized) by caring for his wife for several years as she continued to deteriorate. She never asked him to kill her, and she never suggested that she would be better off dead, but she did say, on several occasions, "I hate my life."

The husband tried to get her into a nursing home, or to change doctors or hospitals, in order to achieve a proper diagnosis with more successful treatment, but she refused. It was his frustration and anger at her refusal that led to his decision that her death was the only alternative.

On examination, he was very open about the fact that she had not asked him to kill her and that he had not considered it until the day that he decided to shoot her to "put her out of her misery." He loaded the gun with two shells, and shot her. He did not give her an overdose of medication, or suffocate her, or kill her in a non-violent manner, but considered only the acute, quick death that he believed would be less painful. He clearly killed her with no malice and with altruism, and did so as a euthanasia procedure rather than cold-blooded murder. He was very disturbed afterward, and clearly had not considered either the consequences or an alternative means of handling a critical situation.

Shortly after the shooting, he called his daughter and told her to call an attorney and the police. He did so because he knew he had done something that was against the law, knew he would be arrested, and knew he would require legal advice and help following the killing of his wife. Even so, he was seen by the defense psychiatrist as not knowing what he was doing was wrong. The defense expert concluded that he later recognized that he had done something wrong, but did not think about it or know it at the time of the shooting.

The prosecution expert saw this more as a mercy killing, without malice, but not as insanity, and did not find evidence for PTSD. He found no evidence for serious dementia that would keep him from knowing what he was doing or knowing that it was wrong. Clearly, he did know that killing his wife was against the law, but he said he felt desperate and had no other alternatives. He, in fact, recognized that he did have alternatives, but they were blocked by her rather than aided by her. Nevertheless, he could have asked for help, gotten her into a nursing home, and spared himself the agony of knowing he had killed her and would be living without her. What he failed to recognize was that even though it was a burden on him (though he denied it), he still took comfort in her presence and her being with him as his companion. After the shooting, he realized how much he missed her and how alone he felt in the world, since he was elderly and many of their friends had died.

The issue here is how does one assess such a vulnerable individual, an elderly man who is charged with killing his wife? One needs to look at all the records, talk to other people who knew him and his wife to determine their relationship, and to work with him in a sympathetic manner, since it is clear that he did not kill her out of jealousy, rage or malice, but, in his own mind, did so with altruism and love. The other side of the story, of course, is that he was also relieving himself of the burden of caring for her, since he had to help her dress and undress, go to the toilet, and help her off the toilet. He was not able to pick her up when she fell, because he was also injured and had no strength in his legs. He was required to call 911 on several occasions to help him get her off the floor when she had fallen. He was embarrassed, he was upset that these events were happening, and felt he had no other recourse.

In preparing a report on this vulnerable individual, one needs to be sensitive to his concerns, his future, and his suffering for the loss of his wife. However, one cannot go to the extreme of believing that he did not know what he was doing since he had no illness that would prevent him from that knowledge or the knowledge that killing his wife was wrong, but one also needs to not go to the other extreme in order to incarcerate him, since he would likely die in jail if found guilty of the homicide of his wife. Thus, the report would need to be sympathetic, balanced, and recommending optimal care for this person, who has never had criminal charges in his 80 years and would likely have a difficult time in a regular prison. Should he be hospitalized or placed in outpatient treatment, and what about relatives who might help care for him? All of these factors must be considered in the disposition of this very difficult and challenging case.

And what about testimony? Should there be a battle of the experts over the question of insanity? Should it be that he would either be acquitted or that he would be found guilty? Either way, he would serve some time in an institution, either a prison (where he probably does not belong and would not do well) or a mental hospital where he would have difficulty fitting in since he lacks serious mental illness. Perhaps the best resolution in this case is for him to have treatment for the depression that he feels for the loss of his wife, and to help him understand what he did and how the issues can be resolved. There is no fear that he will harm anyone else, but there is some concern that he may become suicidal as he realizes how alone and depressed he is. Thus, he may need more protection from himself than protecting others from him.

Ideally, the testimony should be before a sensitive and understanding judge, since a jury would have difficulty parsing out the legal nuances involved in such a challenging and complex case.

It is here that the expert for the prosecution can be helpful to the judge in reaching a decision, not only on the charges, but, more importantly, on the disposition. What will happen to this man? What should happen to him? As the prosecutor has said—Do we want to let him go so that others will see that no punishment occurs when one kills one's wife or husband? The answer is, of course, we do not want to encourage such behavior, but the disposition in this particular case will have little effect on future cases as a deterrent or as an encouragement. People who are faced with desperate situations will not know or remember what happened to this man and will act according to their own morality, ethics, and mental state. Each case must be taken individually and managed for its own specific difficulties and challenges.

When assessing elderly individuals charged with crimes, the forensic assessor must consider the totality of the mental, physical, and social situation. There was a case of a female attorney who killed her parents, because she was psychotic and believed they were suffering, and believed they were asking her to put them to death to relieve their misery. Because of her psychosis, she was found not guilty by reason of insanity (NGRI), and spent many years in the hospital system. It took many years for her to emerge from the system, despite the fact that she was getting on in years and was in her seventies by the time she was released. It was clear that she was not going to harm anyone else and that the object of her violent behavior was only her parents, and that was done for altruistic, psychotic, reasons. Sometimes the system punishes the mentally ill, because of the violence of their behavior and their need for retribution.

Another case involved a physician who killed his wife, and did so when he was legally insane, according to a number of psychiatrists who examined him. However, he was aware, as were his attorneys, that if he were found NGRI, he would go to a hospital for several years, as did the female attorney who killed her parents. He did not wish to go to the hospital for so many years, because of his advancing age, which would amount to a life sentence for him. Instead, he pled to a lesser degree of homicide, that is, voluntary manslaughter, for which he received a brief sentence in prison. He was treated prior to his sentence, and did not require further treatment at that time.

There is also the case of mercy killing, that is, euthanasia, in which one elderly spouse kills the other, because the victim is suffering and "dying anyway." Sometimes, both are in their advanced years, and they agree on a pact that one will kill the ailing person, and then kill him- or herself in a murder-suicide pact. What often happens is that the person who kills their spouse then does not successfully complete their suicide and is charged with the murder of their elderly spouse. How is that person to be handled by the examining forensic mental health expert?

There is also the case of elder abuse by families who care for their elder parents in their home because they cannot afford nursing home care or assisted living. Here the issue is not harm that can be prevented by the forensic expert, but the harm to be prevented in caring for the elderly. Can we, in some way, influence society to provide care for the indigent elderly, who will not be at the mercy of their families who cannot afford to put them in proper institutional care? There is also to be considered the issue of assisted suicide by physicians when the doctor becomes involved to diminish the pain or suffering of an elderly patient.

Kern [3] discusses issues of treatment of the elderly within institutions, similar to the concerns that Isaac Ray had in treating patients over a century ago. My concern in this treatise is more for the vulnerability of the elderly in forensic cases. Many have been abused and harmed by the system, by society in general, and may also be harmed by inappropriate or biased assessments by forensic psychiatrists.

8.3   Other Vulnerable Individuals

What can be said for the elderly can also be said for the mentally retarded, for the underage, and for the seriously mentally ill who do not have the capacity to reason as clearly as the average intelligent adult.

In many of these instances, society has risen to the challenge to mitigate the harm done to vulnerable populations involved in litigation. However, efforts to decriminalize children involved in violent matters have not been that successful. We have attempted, through the juvenile court system, to treat children and adolescents differently from adults and to minimize the harm by not labeling them as criminals. However, we have placed them in facilities where criminal behavior and violence thrive and encourage further violent or criminal behavior in these youngsters when they mature. We have seen these institutions as "training grounds" for future criminal behavior. This is not true in every case, and much effort has gone into modifying and improving the environment in which we place these youngsters. However, much more needs to be done in order to minimize the harm to these vulnerable populations.

8.3.1   *The Mentally Retarded (MR)*

Here we have individuals who may be difficult to interview or examine because of their low IQ, and their difficulty in communicating. It is important for the mental health professional to be able to communicate effectively with the intellectually challenged or developmentally challenged (MR) person. Too often, people speak too rapidly, and the examinee is not properly understood or does not clearly understand what the examiner is talking about. We also have the issue of the mentally retarded and the death penalty, and how we must examine to determine whether the person is sufficiently retarded so as to avoid the death penalty under the Supreme Court Ruling of *Penry v. Lynaugh* (1989) [4].

The mentally retarded may also be taken advantage of in criminal cases, where they are interrogated by the police and information is given to the defendant, who then regurgitates it back unknowingly without thinking about it clearly. Is the individual competent to have confessed? Is the mentally retarded individual competent to stand trial or to be sentenced? These are all issues to consider regarding competency and the mentally retarded.

Siegert and Weiss [5], discuss the issue of competency to stand trial (CST) in defendants who have mental retardation or borderline intellectual functioning. They note this assessment can be difficult when deficits are masked by the type of adaptations seen in many with developmental disabilities. They use validated test instruments and tests measuring receptive and expressive language to augment the clinical interview. The authors note that it is difficult in many of these cases and stress the fact that clinicians conducting these assessments need adequate experience and training in some of the less known psychometric tests before presenting evidence in court. The authors present a case in New Jersey in which the judge accepted the testimony of less experienced experts in order to find the defendant competent. The finding was reversed on appeal. Thus, this case illustrates the need for training and expertise in conducting these assessments, or the result may be harmful to the defendant if the judge accepts the opinion of those who are less well trained.

The authors discuss the appellate court's opinion noting that "the state expert's lack of specific experience with the mentally retarded led her to make errors in evaluating the defendant's competencies in several areas as well as in scoring the CAST-MR."[1] However, the court had no general criticism of the expert's overall competency in the area of CST. The decision was not about the admissibility threshold for expert testimony in this area, note the authors, "Rather, it concerned the relative weight of various experts' opinions and the need for significant experience with this population" [6].

Because people with mental retardation represent a vulnerable population in the criminal justice system, the recommendations of the authors are important in minimizing harm to them. The authors state,

---

[1] Competence Assessment to Stand Trial For Defendants With Mental Retardation.

In addition to our cautionary tale about too casual use of the CAST-MR, we offer the following general points about assessing CST in persons with subnormal intellect:

- *The defendant will try to conceal his or her deficits. Short replies and glibness may function as a defense against exposing areas about which the defendant may feel profound shame.*
- *The defendant may answer in the affirmative, but the responses may have a perseverative quality (acquiescence response set).*
- *The examiner must never accept a simple yes or no, or even many brief replies as a complete response.*
- *Specialized tests of language functioning may be required. Such tests often give a meaningful representation of what a defendant will actually hear or process [7].*

It is important to adhere to these recommendations and guidelines in order to minimize harm to this vulnerable population.

8.3.2   The Severely Mentally Ill

The severely mentally ill individuals are also vulnerable to examination in criminal and civil cases. The schizophrenic or the severely psychotic manic depressive may not be competent to stand trial or to proceed in a civil case. They need to be examined by competent, experienced forensic experts. We may need to determine the mental state of individuals who gave confessions to the police because they were psychotic when, in fact, they were not guilty of the crime. Why do people confess and how do we take care of those who confess out of anxiety or mental illness?

There is the case of a man who spent 18 years on death row for the rape killing of a neighbor woman. He had not killed her, and had resisted the interrogation attempts by the detectives for many hours, but finally, his will was overborne by the police, because he was seriously mentally ill and they were especially skilled at interviewing and interrogating suspects. He said he was told that if he agreed to tell them about killing the woman, they would let him go. He was desperate to go home, and his emotional weakness overrode his logic, which would tell anyone that if one confesses to a murder, the police are not going to let him go. However, he did confess, was confused, and was convicted. He had less than effective assistance of counsel and was given the death penalty. It was only on appeal, with the help of DNA testing, that showed that he could not have committed the act for which he was deceived to confess.

The attorneys, following his release from prison, asked why he would or how he could confess to a crime that he did not commit. The question arose in the civil case for damages by the state for having forced an innocent man to confess, and then taken 18 years of his life under false circumstances.

It is not unusual for people to want to get out of a very difficult, tense, and frightening, if not extremely stressful, situation. The mentally ill and the mentally retarded are especially sensitive and vulnerable under such circumstances [8]. As Janofsky [9] points out, the courts have upheld and allowed the interrogators to be deceptive and to lie to the suspects in order to get a confession. The mentally ill and mentally retarded are especially vulnerable under these circumstances and, of course, the mental health examiners must not utilize similar methods when assessing such defendants.

Another case involved a man in the military who was witness to a knife killing outside a bar while stationed in Germany many years ago. He was handed the knife and helped bury it to obstruct justice and avoid arrest of his associate, who did the stabbing. He had difficulty sleeping, with nightmares, for the next several weeks, and when the CID came to interrogate him, he immediately confessed to the crime, as he had begun to feel especially guilty for hiding the evidence. He was arrested on the charges and was assessed for his mental state and his ability to confess to a crime that he did not commit. It was determined that he was psychotic and was having delusions about guilt feelings for other behaviors in the past that were exaggerated in his mind. He believed he required punishment and confessed to this crime so that he would be punished. He was also hearing voices and seeing visions of the victim in this case, with blood on his hands. It was determined that he was psychotic and that his confession was not valid, but was based on delusional ideation.

This is a case in which the individual may have been harmed by the system and his own feelings of guilt, because he was vulnerable and seriously mentally ill. It was only through intervention by proper forensic psychiatric assessment and testing that led to his being released from arrest for a crime that he did not commit. The system may not be sensitive to the seriousness of mental illness with respect to confessions or stability to stand trial and should depend upon accurate and objective forensic psychiatric assessment to achieve justice and minimize harm to vulnerable individuals.

With respect to the seriously mentally ill, there is also the case of the mass murderer who received a death penalty for killing several people in one night. He spent 25 years on death row, and continued to deteriorate over that time, becoming psychotic, with delusions, hallucinations, and multiple somatic symptoms. He was assessed for competency to be executed, and was found to be incompetent to be put to death. He did not understand the reasons for his death penalty and was not able to competently understand his role within the system.

The examination of this individual was quite difficult, because of his violent nature and his psychotic delusional system that affected his ability to communicate. Finding such an individual competent (as the prosecution experts did) would have been harmful to him had the judge agreed with their assessment rather than the findings of the defense psychiatrists who clearly found him incompetent to be executed.

It was my understanding, from the defense attorneys, that their client was so severely mentally ill that he could not effectively communicate with them or with his mental health experts. The defense was surprised to learn that the prosecution mental health experts reached the conclusion that the defendant was competent under those circumstances. The judge, observing the defendant himself, agreed with the experts who found him incompetent. The defendant was then sent to the hospital for further treatment, and the final adjudication was that he was incompetent to be executed, and his sentence was commuted. Finding him competent to be executed could have led to his execution. Balance and objectivity are required in these special cases to prevent further harm to vulnerable individuals.

8.3.3   Children Vulnerable to Violence

We turn briefly to the issue of children who are vulnerable to being killed by their parents, sometimes known as neonaticide, infanticide or filicide [10]. There is a case of a woman who killed her six-year-old daughter because she believed that she was dying a painful death from cancer. In fact, she had no cancer, but had a chronic illness and was not in pain as she had believed in her delusional psychotic condition. She felt the doctors had missed the diagnosis and that she could perceive the suffering in her daughter where others could not.

She killed her in a most humane way so that she would not suffer, and believed that she had done the right thing. In the course of the evaluation, her attorney asked that I not discuss her case with her husband, who was not sympathetic with her inasmuch as he was grieving the loss of his daughter and the "betrayal" of his wife. I felt it was important to talk to her husband to get his particular point of view, and also for him to understand the dynamics of her mental illness that led to the tragedy. She wanted me to speak to her husband in spite of the fact that her attorney had asked that I not do so. Her husband had planned to divorce her because of her violence toward their daughter and his fear that she may harm the other children.

I waited until after the trial to discuss the matter with her husband, who wanted to know more about her and why this tragedy occurred. I was able to have her send a signed release of information form so that I could talk with her husband and explain to him what had occurred. He appeared to understand her problem and why she was found legally not responsible. He also felt she was mentally out of control and, therefore, not responsible. However, he continued to believe that at some level, she had to be held responsible for the death of their daughter and, indeed, she was. It was her body that had killed her daughter even though her mind was distorted and her beliefs were delusional and psychotic. Part of her rehabilitation was his writing to her telling her he understood her condition and was willing, at some time in the future, to forgive her. She continued to hope for a reconciliation and looked forward to her treatment knowing that it would take several years before she would be released. She continued to see her older children, who regarded her as their mother and needed to see her regularly. Her husband continued to be supportive, but he decided to move on with his life.

This example is one where one does not only "do no harm" or minimizes the harm, the non-maleficence, but also shows that one can be beneficent in the handling of very difficult cases by active intervention.

Clearly, young children are at the mercy of their parents, who may kill for a number of reasons. Elsewhere, I have discussed the killing of children by mothers for various reasons [11], depending on the age of the children and the dynamics of the mother's mental illness. For example, I noted some mothers killed their newborns because they were not aware that they were pregnant, had denied their pregnancy or were overwhelmed at the time of the birth of the child when they are alone, vulnerable, and under great stress. Older children may be killed because mother has a delusion that father is going to torture them or harm them, worse than death, so the mother, before killing herself, decides to kill her children to spare them the suffering she anticipates coming from their father.

There is also the case of Andrea Yates [12], who killed her children because of a psychotic delusional belief and hallucinations.

In another case, a man killed his two children in order to spare them the suffering of being converted from Judaism to Christianity when his wife and he divorced and she decided to marry a Christian man, move away and raise the children as Christian. He had his last visitation with the children and decided that life was not worth living. He would kill himself and the children so they would not be converted and thus not go to heaven, as he envisioned it. He put the gas on at home, when they were sleeping. They died, but he did not. He was tried and convicted for their murders.

I had examined this man for the prosecution and found that he was not legally insane, because he had a belief system that was not delusional, but it was extreme. When it came to examining him for the death penalty, I told the prosecutors that I felt there were enough mitigating circumstances because of his extreme emotional condition that clouded his judgment and enabled him to carry out his homicidal and suicidal intent. He was spared the death penalty and is currently serving two life sentences.

I use this example to illustrate that even though working for the prosecution and finding no evidence for insanity, one may still find sufficient mitigating circumstances that would not warrant the death penalty.

These examples are given to illustrate the vulnerability of children who are at the mercy of their parents and may be killed for any number of reasons. They also illustrate the vulnerability of the people convicted of killing their children. Many have biases toward those who kill, torture, or abuse children, and this bias may emerge in the course of examining parents or others who kill children. It behooves the forensic psychiatric examiner to be as sensitive, objective and unbiased as possible when conducting a forensic examination of these defendants as well. We do not want our bias to harm the parents who kill children when the parents may be deluded, misinformed, or malicious. In many ways, they have already been harmed by their own behavior and need not be further harmed during the forensic examination.

8.3.4   Individuals with Disability

Many years ago, I served as a member of the task force of the American Psychiatric Association on the use and misuse of psychiatric diagnoses in the legal process. A paper was published in the Bulletin of AAPL in 1992, delineating some of the concerns of the task force [13]. Initially, the article discusses the sources of misunderstanding and confusion, indicating the conceptual distance between diagnoses and functional capacities. There are a number of psychiatrists who tend to focus on diagnosis and attribute legal capacities to a medical diagnosis rather than specifying what limitations they have as a result of that diagnosis. For example, there are psychiatrists who believe that all schizophrenics are not competent to stand trial or would be found NGRI just because they have a psychosis and do not always deal with reality. The authors state,

> When diagnoses are used to infer functional impairments in a global, categorical fashion, it is a disservice performed to the courts, to the psychiatric profession, and to patients. The court cannot test the premises used by the evaluating psychiatrists in reaching their conclusions ... The court is deprived of essential data about the relationship of disorder to impairment and dysfunction ... When diagnoses are used in this way, they are of little value and in some cases can result in confusion and judicial error [13].

For example, the authors note,

> Patients who have such a disorder may be falsely assumed to have certain disabilities. Such assumptions may diminish their employability or acceptance in a variety of social situations. When participants who are observers of the legal process have had experiences at variance with that expressed by the experts, the credibility of the profession may be undermined and patients may face new forms of prejudice and stigmatization [13].

Consistent with the assessment of individuals who have disabilities, are those who are assessed for competency. Often, the examination of an individual is for his or her ability or competency to perform various tasks either in the legal setting, in their work, or in general.

Gutheil and Bursztajn [14] note the importance of assessing competency and how subtle forms of incompetency may be missed. Their article suggests strategies for clinicians in conducting assessments of subtle competency in legal matters. The importance of this paper is that it presents those cases in which competency may be missed, especially when assessed by unsophisticated, non-forensically trained psychiatrists in consultation and liaison work. For example, someone is refusing treatment and may be incompetent to do so, or an individual is unwilling or unable to consent to a surgical procedure.

This concept is extremely important, especially in light of the critical papers of Morris *et al.* [15] and Perlin *et al.* [16] who question the competency of psychiatrists to assess competency in legal matters. They show by their research that psychiatrists vary widely in their assessment of individuals for competency procedures. Their studies are especially important in demonstrating the lack of agreement among forensic psychiatrists in their assessment procedures and conclusions. We need to develop more accurate measures of assessment to become more efficient, effective, and scientific in our approach in order to minimize further harm to those we examine and assess. This is especially true for the vulnerable populations outlined in this chapter: the elderly, the mentally retarded, and the severely mentally disabled.

8.4 Summary

This chapter is primarily about minimizing the harm caused by the forensic examiners to vulnerable individuals. The harm that can be caused to these people by the system is clear, and is well illustrated by case examples, but we, forensic mental health experts, do not need to aggravate the harm that is inherent in the system, especially to these vulnerable individuals.

References

1. Birnbaum, M. (1960) The right to treatment. *American Bar Association Journal*, **46**, 499.
2. Perlin, M.L. (1989) *Mental Disability Law: Civil and Criminal*, The Michie Company, Charlottesville.
3. Kern, S. (1990) Protecting the rights of the elderly, in *Ethical Practice in Psychiatry and the Law* (eds. R. Rosner and R. Weinstock), Plenum Press, New York, pp. 307–12.
4. *Penry v. Lynaugh*, 492 US 302, (1989).
5. Siegert, M. and Weiss, K.J. (2007) Who is an expert? Competency evaluations and mental retardation and borderline intelligence. *Journal of the American Academy of Psychiatry and the Law*, **35**, 346–49.
6. See Ref. [5], p. 348.
7. See Ref. [5], p. 349.
8. Weiss, K.J. (2003) Confessions and expert testimony. *Journal of the American Academy of Psychiatry and the Law*, **31**, 451–58.
9. Janofsky, J. (2006) Lies and coercion: Why psychiatrists should not participate in police and intelligence interrogations. *Journal of the American Academy of Psychiatry and the Law*, **34**(4), 472–8.
10. Resnick, P.J. (1969) Child murder by parents: a psychiatric review of filicide. *The American Journal of Psychiatry*, **126**, 325–34.
11. Sadoff, R.L. (1995) Mothers who kill their children. *Psychiatric Annals*, **25**, 10.
12. *Yates v. State*, 171 SW 3d 215, (Tex. App. 2005).
13. Halleck, S.L., Hoge, S.K., Miller, R.D. *et al.* (1992) The use of psychiatric diagnoses in the legal process: Task force report of the American Psychiatric Association. *Bulletin of the American Academy of Psychiatry and the Law*, **20**, 481–99.
14. Gutheil, T.G. and Bursztajn, H. (1996) Clinicians' guidelines for assessing and presenting subtle forms of patient incompetence in legal settings. *The American Journal of Psychiatry*, **143**(8), 1020–3.
15. Morris, G.H., Haroun, A.M., and Naimark, D. (2004) Assessing competency competently: toward a rational standard for competency to stand trial assessments. *Journal of the American Academy of Psychiatry and the Law*, **32**, 231–45.
16. Perlin, M.L., Champine, P., Dlugacz, H.A., and Connell, M. (2008) *Competence in the Law: From Legal Theory to Clinical Application*, John Wiley & Sons, Inc., New York.

9 Victims and Predators of Sexual Violence

Robert L. Sadoff

University of Pennsylvania School of Medicine, Philadelphia, USA

9.1 Introduction

Victims of sexual crimes may be vulnerable individuals when it comes to forensic psychiatric examinations. The women who are victims of rape or aggravated sexual assault can be further traumatized by insensitive psychiatric examiners for the defense who wish to "get all the details" of the sexual behavior of the defendant. They will make the victim go through the excruciating details of her traumatic experience, having her relive the horrendous attack on her and the emotional as well as physical consequences of the harm that was caused during the assault.

Interviewers may be sincere in "seeking truth and justice," especially if the defendant claims the sexual behavior was consensual and not forced. They may question the victim in order to determine the consistency of her statements and the credibility of her accusations. Alternatively, they may be curious due to their own psychodynamics about the specifics of the assault or they may be sadistic in wishing to have the victim suffer even further. They also may have a little bit of all of the above. We do not always know why people choose the professions they do and why they select particular areas of their work that seem to give them more pleasure. Could the examiner interview the victim in a sensitive manner, without all of the gory details? Would that be fair to their client, and would they actually be striving for objectivity and seeking truth and justice?

9.2 In Civil Cases

In civil cases where young women sue for damages after claiming to have been sexually abused by their employers or by fellow employees, they may be subject

Ethical Issues in Forensic Psychiatry: Minimizing Harm by Robert L. Sadoff
© 2011 John Wiley & Sons, Ltd

to examination by forensic mental health experts. There are a series of tests that psychologists give to victims of sexual abuse to determine whether they meet the criteria for PTSD caused by the sexual assault, and there are tests given to the perpetrators to determine if they are sexual psychopaths or sexually violent predators (SVPs).

Just as we have seen in child psychiatry that fathers of daughters can be falsely accused of sexually violating their children, so can employers or fellow employees be falsely accused for political, social, or economic reasons. Just because a plaintiff in a civil case accuses someone of sexually abusing them, does not mean that it has actually happened. We must remember the spate of cases a couple of decades ago where young women with eating disorders and other behavioral disorders or depression were deemed by their therapists to have been sexually abused as children and they needed to remember what had happened. In the course of therapy for a number of these young women, memories bubbled up to the surface and accusations were made against parents, siblings, neighbors, physicians, and others who had contact with the young girl as she was growing and developing.

9.2.1   Case Examples

One case that was extreme involved a 27-year-old woman who initially accused her father of having sex with her between the ages of five and seven, and then she included her brothers, her uncles, and her physician. She initially sued her father with the help of a female attorney, who believed her accusations and accompanied her to the examination that I performed at the request of her father's attorney. Her attorney was berating me for having artwork in my office that was insulting to her client and "harmful" to her, because some of my sculpture showed intact families and some of the paintings were also of close-knit families. On the second visit, the attorney returned with a camera to photograph these "offensive" pieces of art that I "deliberately" had in my office in order to offend her client. She was going to show them in court to indicate my bias and my hostility toward her client. The case never developed, however, because the client continued to include every male she had ever contacted as having sexually abused her. Even her attorney began to doubt her credibility and decided she had no case and left her client.

I had to ask myself whether my artwork was indeed offensive, and should I remove it from my office, or was this another ploy by the plaintiff to intimidate or to "rack up points" for her side? The artwork remains three decades later without anyone else considering it to be offensive, but rather to be peaceful, comforting, and reassuring.

I have examined several dozen adult "victims" of sexual abuse by their religious mentors, including priests, rabbis, ministers, and others. Mostly, I consulted with the Catholic churches in order to help defend the claims that were brought well after the statute of limitations had ended. The issue was whether or not the victims recognized that they had been sexually abused and that the symptoms they experienced were caused by the abuse which was harmful to them. Most indicated that they had not considered what the priest had done to them as sexually offensive and did not believe they were harmed, but rather that they were special and were singled out by their religious leaders for special treatment. Although many claimed that they had no knowledge of being abused, it was determined through collateral interviews and other sources that they had complained of the abuse to others many years before and could have filed a complaint in court had they chosen to do so. They were not so mentally ill or retarded that they could not have filed.

These individuals are all vulnerable within the legal system and need to be examined with sensitivity and concern even when working for the defense. I was moved by the numbers of people who had been so abused and the effect it had upon them and their lives. Some were able to marry, others left the church, and most continued to have some psychological effect that was damaging and harmful to them. In my opinion, one had to be extremely sensitive when conducting the examination so as not to further harm these vulnerable individuals.

9.3 Sexual Perpetrators

Similarly, the perpetrator of sexual offenses is also a potentially vulnerable individual, especially with the recent Megan's Law [1], where they would be seen in many states as an SVP. Individuals labeled as SVPs have to report their address and their status when they are released from prison and must register in their locality for the rest of their lives. In other jurisdictions, the registration can be obligatory for 10 years, or other limited period.[1]

In considering the perpetrators, we have to also consider what happens to sex offenders in prison. There is a hierarchy of criminal behavior, with murder at the top and pedophilia at the bottom. Nobody loves a "short eyes," one who has sexually abused children. Pedophiles do not do well in prison when the nature of their crime is known. They are often victimized by other inmates and taunted and teased and/or raped repeatedly. Prison officials are sensitive to the diagnoses and problems of their inmates and tend to separate those who are more vulnerable and likely to be assaulted. They are often placed in a special housing unit known as "protective custody."

There appears to be a natural antipathy toward sex offenders, especially those who violate children. Many people have an inherent bias against such individuals, and it should be noted that even forensic psychiatrists may act out against such individuals by preparing harmful reports and making recommendations for punishment rather than treatment.

Thus, both the victim of sex offenses and the perpetrator are vulnerable individuals within the system, especially when confronting forensic psychiatrists who may not be aware of their own biases. I have seen too often that the victim of sexual offense is believed without corroboration, and the plaintiff's expert in civil

---

[1] Alaska Statute Sections 12.63.010 (d) (1), 12.63.020 (a) (2) 15 years or if "convicted of an aggravated sex offense or of two or more sex offenses, he must register for life . . . ." Connecticut General Statute Section 54-251 (2008). Minnesota Statute Section 243.166 (2008). NJ Statute Section 2C:7-2 (2008). New York C.L.S. Correc. Section 168-h (2008). Pennsylvania 42 Pa.C.S. Section 9795.1.

cases of sexual assault accepts the plaintiff's words without question and states that the symptoms are clearly caused by the sexual assault (whether or not it ever occurred). On the other hand, there are those who will find accused sexual offenders guilty in their own mind and accept that they are in need of treatment and/or punishment because they are sex offenders, which means they have both negative aspects, the sexual violent behavior, and the violation of criminal laws.

There was recently a case determined by the Supreme Court [2] to not impose the death penalty on a man who had sexually raped a young girl and then killed her. Commentators were lined up on both sides, including those who were totally against the death penalty hailing the decision, and those who were mostly against the death penalty, but stating they could not understand the court not imposing death in this case because it involved a sexual assault on a youngster and then the murder of his victim. There appears to be an inherent fear of the sexually violent person who needs to be controlled and punished despite the fact that he or she may be seriously mentally ill, with the illness causing their violent sexual behavior.

9.4 Boundary Violations

Gutheil and Brodsky [3] have discussed the difference between boundary crossings and boundary violations when it comes to sexual behavior. They note that boundary crossings occur frequently in the course of therapy and may be ethically in question, but are not criminal, nor are they the subject of malpractice suits. However, boundary violations such as sexually touching a female patient without consent (or even with consent) is forbidden and may be the subject of three major concerns for the perpetrating psychiatrist. First, he may lose his license and his position within his professional organizations. Secondly, he may be sued civilly for damages to his patient if it can be proven that he did that of which he is accused, and the behavior charged led to damage to the patient. Third, he may be charged criminally with rape or sexual assault, depending on the circumstances.

Gutheil also points out that the most common diagnosis for women who have been the victims of boundary violations is borderline personality disorder [4]. He also notes that most of those who falsely accuse their therapist of boundary violations are also diagnosed with borderline personality disorder. It behooves the therapist to be very cautious when treating a borderline person not to have any boundary crossings, let alone boundary violations. The borderline may interpret a boundary crossing as a violation and take legal action. In those cases, the treating psychiatrist becomes a vulnerable individual as well.

I have presented elsewhere in this book the case of a woman who had accused her psychiatrist of boundary violations and sexually attacking her. She had lied in court about my examination, but fortunately, I was chaperoned by her expert, who was my former teacher and mentor. To his credit and my good fortune, he testified in court that his patient had lied about me, as he was present and his "former student was nothing but professional."

The message here is that the vulnerable forensic examiner conducting an assessment involving a borderline personality disorder or an antisocial personality disorder should take precaution not to be attacked verbally or physically during or after the examination. This is another example of the vulnerability of the forensic psychiatric examiner and how harm to the examiner can be minimized with care and caution.

With respect to sexual accusations, Billick [5], discusses the problem of accusations by children of sexual abuse and the effect on prosecutors. He states that for the longest time he tried to convince pediatricians that they should take seriously the sexual abuse allegations made by children. He states now the pendulum has swung, and he tries to convince prosecutors that children's comments are not always accurate. He recalls a case involving the allegation of inappropriate touching: the grandfather was urologically incapable of achieving a penile erection, but was convicted of criminal sexual abuse, including penile penetration on his granddaughter on allegations arising during the time that she was psychotic and hospitalized in a psychiatric facility. (This example demonstrates the vulnerability of the elderly as they may be caught up in the system and harmed when others lie about them, despite their physical incapabilities.)

Billick [5] notes another instance when a father took over the daily feeding and hygiene needs of his two pre-school daughters. At that time, his wife was hospitalized, undergoing surgery and rehabilitation. Allegations of inappropriate touching were made, and it seemed obvious that the miscommunications arose from his inexperienced bathing techniques. The prosecutor, however, isolated these children in foster placement and kept both parents from them while the children were prepared for court. The potential for contaminated memory in rehearsing testimony was so great in these young children that Billick contends their testimony should have been precluded. He questioned whether the alleged sexual abuse was worse than the separation of the children from their mother for nearly a year at such a tender age. He states, "Our solutions both temporary and permanent, must be tempered by the severity of the causative abuse of actions."

Billick tells us the world is not perfect, and neither is our psychiatric science. He states, "We must learn to accept some ambiguity and uncertainty. For example, we cannot expect an autistic child who cannot remember what she had for breakfast to recall accurately whether she was sexually molested by her father" [5]. Yet, he states he has seen social welfare workers attempt to have autistic children testify under oath.

In cases of abuse of minors, Billick asks,

Do we really want to have overkill in our protection of the child? It simply is not appropriate to take an otherwise well adjusted happy autistic child from her lifelong home and nuclear family when she may have been the victim of at most minor sexual abuse. This is particularly true, given the nature of autistic children and sexual behaviors when the abuse is most likely self-inflicted or caused by a pubescent male sibling, rather than the father (who is the focus of the investigation).

Further, he states, "We must balance in our weighing of the competitive traumas the disorder versus the cure. Oncologists do this daily, but we are not yet so experienced."

Billick closes with a philosophical concern and an admonition for all of us,

We yearn to have answers and to have solutions. We want to prosecute the wrongdoers and protect the innocent. Children need us to be vigilant in identifying and correcting abusive environments. But the children also need us to be mature and to use judgment and balance in our assessments and in our recommendation for corrective actions [5].

I inserted this material here rather than in Chapter 7 because it has more to do with sexual offenses and vulnerability than just with children. We may generalize, from Billick's comments, beyond children as victims, and state that we want to "prosecute the wrongdoers and protect the innocent." But we also should note, as Billick states, that the victims need us to be mature and to use judgment and balance in our assessments and in our recommendations. His comments and suggestions are in keeping with the ethical guidelines of AAPL, and if we adhere to them, we will minimize harm not only to the victims of sexual abuse, but also to the perpetrators (some of whom may be innocent).

References

1. Megan's Law, NJ Statute Section 2C:7-2, (2008).
2. See *Stansbury v. California*, 511 US 318, 114 S. Ct. 1526, 128 L. Ed. 2d. 293, (1994).
3. Gutheil, T.G. and Brodsky, A. (2008) *Preventing Boundary Violations in Clinical Practice*, Guilford Press, New York.
4. Gutheil, T.G. (1992) Approaches to forensic assessment of false claims of sexual misconduct by therapists. *Bulletin of the American Academy of Psychiatry and the Law*, **20**, 289–96.
5. Billick, S.B. (2001) Preserving balance in forensic psychiatry. *Journal of the American Academy of Psychiatry and the Law*, **29**, 372–3.

10 Immigrants: A Vulnerable Population

Solange Margery Bertoglia

Thomas Jefferson University Hospital, Philadelphia, USA

10.1 Introduction

According to the United States Census Bureau's 2008 American Community Survey, 12.5% of the total United States population are immigrants [1]. The numbers tend to vary depending on whether illegal immigrants are estimated and included, and whether other groups are also accounted for (e.g., asylum seekers, temporary visa holders, etc.). In this chapter, the term immigrant will be used to refer to persons who were not United States citizens at birth (including: naturalized citizens, lawful permanent residents, refugees, and asylees, persons on temporary visas, and illegal immigrants). Official organizations, such as the United Nations [2,3] and the United States Department of Homeland Security [4], have specific definitions to differentiate some of these groups.

Immigration can be a stressful life circumstance. Some immigrants have escaped war, political persecution, and extreme poverty. Further psychological stress can result from the process of immigration and integration to a new country. Children born to immigrants will inherit some of their parents' adversities because of their creed, race, name, and so on. Immigrants are often lumped together into groups based on race, language, religious affiliation, or other random characteristics. In reality, what probably defines a group best is its ethnic background. "Ethnicity can be measured using a variety of concepts, including ethnic ancestry or origin, ethnic identity, cultural origins, nationality, race, color, minority status, tribe, language, religion, or various combinations of these concepts" [5]. For the purpose of this chapter, ethnicity refers to a common culture, creed, and mores and not necessarily to common language or race.

Ethical Issues in Forensic Psychiatry: Minimizing Harm by Robert L. Sadoff
© 2011 John Wiley & Sons, Ltd

Despite the challenges that immigrants face and their need for mental health care, they might not get this care for several reasons, including: fear that it might affect their residency status or lead to deportation if they are illegal immigrants [6,7], lack of insurance or other resources, negative cultural perception toward mental health, or a more somatic-oriented manifestation of mental illness.

This chapter will describe how immigrants constitute a vulnerable population in the context of forensic evaluations. There are many other aspects in which this population's vulnerability could be discussed (e.g., correctional setting, understanding of the Miranda warning, jury bias, bias in the sentencing process, etc.) but this chapter will be limited to the forensic evaluation itself. It will elaborate further on cases and studies pertaining to Hispanic Americans, and Arab and Muslim Americans.

10.2   Forensic Evaluation of Immigrants

Forensic psychiatrists are often called upon to evaluate immigrants in several different contexts. Forensic psychiatrists can be asked to do asylum evaluations [8,9] or evaluations for waiver of deportation for a permanent resident ("green card" holder) who has committed a crime [9]. In both, the cultural and immigration histories are a fundamental part of the interview. On the other hand, there are many other criminal and civil evaluations in which the impact of the ethnic background can be easily overlooked.

10.2.1   Evaluee of a Different Ethnic Background

The usual case scenario is that of an immigrant being evaluated by a forensic evaluator that does not share the evaluee's ethnic background. The forensic examiner should be aware of the particular vulnerability of the evaluee in this situation. Four important areas that can lead to a biased, incomplete, or erroneous evaluation are: language barrier, countertransference toward the evaluee's ethnicity, ignorance about the evaluee's ethnicity, and evaluee's transference.

10.2.1.1   Language Barrier

Language barrier is the most obvious problem when evaluating someone from a different ethnicity. Interpreters are of great help, yet their degree of training varies and this affects the quality of their work. Frequently, institutions use their bilingual staff as interpreters, despite their lack of training because they are easily available. Even in the case of well-trained interpreters or well-intended staff members, they may not be familiar with the evaluee's dialect or worse, they might not readily admit to this. This language gap becomes a disadvantage for the immigrant, whose narrative might be altered or "lost in translation." Vasquez and Javier showed that the most frequent errors made by untrained Spanish-speaking interpreters are: omission, addition, condensation, substitution, and role exchange [10].

There are other disadvantages for an immigrant who does not speak the language spoken in court. For example, in many immigration courts the interpretation is provided for the immigrant's testimony and questions to the immigrant, but there might not be simultaneous interpretation of the other witnesses' testimonies, arguments between counsel and the judge's statements [11].

10.2.1.2   Countertransference toward the Evaluee's Ethnicity

Because ethnicity is comprised of so many characteristics [5] it allows for multiple sources of negative countertransference, including nationality, race, and religion. The evaluator's bias can arise from a personal, familial, or national experience or be the result of learned stereotypes. Whatever the reason might be, countertransference can affect the course of the interview and might have an impact on the opinion. This can be a problem in criminal cases, in which defendants might have already lost sympathy because of being charged for a criminal act. "Sometimes, antisocial personality disorder is loosely diagnosed without following *DSM-IV* criteria in individuals an examiner does not like if the individual has committed an illegal act" [12]. Negative countertransference toward an immigrant could also affect the outcome of civil cases, such as immigration cases, custody battles [13], disability cases, and civil commitment [13] among others.

Bias can worsen as a response to current political and financial affairs. This is true for Arab- and Muslim-Americans since the events of September, 11, 2001: " . . . failure of government leaders to speak out on a sustained basis against discrimination, coupled with the Justice Department's aggressive immigration initiatives, sent a message to individuals and companies that discrimination against Arabs and Muslims was acceptable . . ." [14]. This bias has been reflected in the often overly quick "terrorist" implication in cases involving Arab, Muslims, or Middle Eastern immigrants [15].

Evaluators can also have a positive countertransference toward an immigrant. This can be because of the immigrant's particular ethnic group or because of the particular circumstances that the immigrant has endured, such as trauma and torture [16].

10.2.1.3   Ignorance about the Evaluee's Ethnicity

The research done on the evaluee's ethnicity frequently amounts to a close-ended question about race or nationality and a short statement about it in the developmental history. Many cases would benefit from a more in-depth look into the evaluee's ethnic background. For example, in asylum evaluations an evaluator must learn about the situation in the evaluee's country of origin. Lack of information can lead to an evaluator's failure to consider common traumatic events experienced by immigrants escaping that country [17]. It is also important to understand the ethnic background "since culture shapes personal identity, emotional responses, and patterns of reasoning . . . (which can) . . . influence motivation and intent . . ." [18]. Lack of information regarding an immigrant's ethnic background and cultural mores can make it difficult to understand his or her views on issues such as corporal punishment, domestic violence [12], custody, age for sexual consent, and so on. This does not imply that an immigrant would be exculpated because of ignorance of the host country laws or for putting his or her own ethnic perceptions above the law. It is, however, a point of consideration in understanding how the immigrant's statements or actions might be better understood within his or her ethnic background.

In other cases, an evaluator might not be familiar with how ethnic backgrounds can influence the manifestation of psychiatric symptoms. For example, Hispanics who experience stress, particularly those with a diagnosis of depression, might have multiple somatic symptoms (more than their Anglo counterparts) [19]. An evaluator might misdiagnose the evaluee with somatization disorder or malingering instead of the recent development of depression and anxiety, which can then affect the evaluee's mental stress claim [12].

Ignoring the implications of the evaluee's ethnic background can lead to many other opportunities for mistakes by the evaluators to affect the immigrant's case. Ignorance of ethnic differences in body language, personal space, and eye contact could be misinterpreted as reflecting a lack of cooperativeness or the presence of a personality trait. An evaluator might also overlook how the roles of gender in society can differ according to the ethnic background. An immigrant might react differently to a male versus a female evaluator. This difference in response might lead to an erroneous interpretation of the immigrant's personality or attitude.

In addition, not knowing about the immigrants' perception of the legal system and how it works can undermine the accuracy of the evaluation. This does not mean that immigrants should be judged by the laws of their country of origin or should claim ignorance of the host country's law as a defense; however, it should be a factor in understanding the case. For example, for some immigrants it might be particularly difficult to understand that a mental health professional can play a non-confidential role. Another example is that of evaluations for competency to stand trial where the concept of admission of guilt to get a "good deal" might be particularly challenging to an immigrant who feels he or she is being "railroaded" [9]. The immigrant's views of the legal system can become even more challenging when the laws of the country of origin come from a religious ideology. Islamic law has its own way of dealing with divorce, child custody, criminal responsibility, compensation of damages, and so on [20]. In the mind of some Muslim immigrants adhering to such law is not only related to following secular laws, it is also about following the word of God.

10.2.1.4　Evaluee's Transference

An immigrant's decision of where to migrate might be less of a deliberate personal choice and more of a decision based on geographical closeness, assistance of relatives, political reasons, and so on. As such, the immigrant's perception of the host country and its habitants can vary. An immigrant might perceive the evaluator as part of a dominant group from which he or she feels victimized or stereotyped. Even a well-intentioned question about a cultural explanation of a belief might feel condescending to an immigrant.

On the other hand, the evaluator can be seen as belonging to a group that will not judge, might sympathize, or even protect the immigrant. This is particularly true in matters that can lead to cultural alienation of the immigrant from his or her own ethnic group. This was the author's experience when doing a civil commitment evaluation on a Pakistani American young woman who had attempted suicide because her traditional Muslim parents were arranging her marriage. She explained how the suicide attempt and the commitment to a psychiatric institution would result in rejection from her community and shame for her family. She spontaneously mentioned she was glad she was not evaluated by someone of her same background as she would feel judged.

10.2.2   *Evaluee of the Same or Similar Ethnic Background*

It is naïve to think that using an evaluator of the same or similar ethnic group to the evaluee will solve all problems. An evaluator from the same or similar background of the evaluee can have some of the same challenges posed to an evaluator of the majority group.

10.2.2.1   *Language Barrier*

As interpreters, native language evaluators are limited by the multiple dialects of a language. One added possibility of bias can come from recognition of an accent. An accent can allow an evaluator to determine the evaluee's nationality or region of birth. For evaluators from an immigrant group, a dialect can point to a region or country that has its own particular stereotypes that go beyond the more general stereotypes created by majority groups.

10.2.2.2   *Countertransference toward the Evaluee's Ethnicity*

An evaluator from a minority group can feel connected to his or her ethnic background and might have a positive countertransference toward an evaluee from the same or similar background. Evaluators who are immigrants themselves might relate to some of the evaluee's experiences and struggles. This is easily implied as the rule by majority groups who might see similar ethnic groups as having friendly relationships, but this does not hold true in many cases. For example, an institution or mediator can have good intentions in choosing an evaluator with the same or similar background as the evaluee. In reality, an evaluator might belong to a country which has been at war or at least in conflict with that of the evaluee. Even if the evaluator and evaluee share a nationality, the evaluator might find out that the evaluee belongs to an opposing religious or political group in a country torn by civil war. The countertransference can be profound if the evaluator or the evaluator's family endured persecution or torture by the evaluee's ethnic group. There are multiple other reasons why an evaluator from the same or similar background might be less than sympathetic to an immigrant. For example, the evaluator might feel that if he or she went through similar immigration circumstances without getting involved in crime or needing disability for mental illness, then the evaluee should have also, thus impacting the evaluation process.

An evaluator could even be publicly judged by evaluating someone of similar or the same background. An Arab- and Muslim-American evaluator whose opinion favors an Arab and Muslim evaluee, especially in immigration cases, can be publicly blamed for conspiring with terrorists [21]. This perception opens a possibility of bias for Arab- and Muslim-American evaluators who might consciously or unconsciously feel the need to appear less preferential toward their own ethnicity.

10.2.2.3   Ignorance about the Evaluee's Ethnicity

Nuances within ethnic backgrounds are diverse and it is a mistake to assume that an evaluator of the same or similar ethnicity is an expert on the immigrant's ethnic background and culture just because they share a language, phenotype, or even country of origin. For example, an evaluator who was born, raised, and studied in an urban setting might know little about the beliefs and customs of the rural people or indigenous people of his or her country. In some cases, the evaluator might have a mistaken assumption of expertise and undermine the need for further learning about the evaluee's specific ethnic background. Furthermore, the evaluee "may withhold key cultural information helpful to the case due to a belief that the psychiatrists of the same ethnic group would necessarily already have that knowledge or might disapprove of certain motivations or actions" [12].

10.2.2.4   Evaluee's Transference

As expected, an evaluee's transference toward an evaluator from the same or similar ethnic background can be positive or negative. Negative feelings can come from various sources, including race, accent, and even socioeconomic status. On the other hand, a positive transference can be too "seductive." An evaluee faced with an evaluator of the same or similar background might "open up" easily and put aside the non-confidentiality disclosure [22].

10.3   Misuse of Ethnic Knowledge

There have been concerns about how cultural or ethnic knowledge is used. For example, it has been argued that individuals can manipulate cultural factors to create bogus defenses [23]. Some point out that allowing immigrants to claim non-responsibility by a cultural defense violates fundamental fairness [24] and that cultural factors can be taken into consideration for diminished responsibility but not as a separate type of defense [25].

In its most harmful way, ethnic knowledge could be applied in intelligence interrogations to find out what would cause the most psychological stress to people of a given background. This is a concern since psychiatrists and psychologists had a "systematic role in developing and executing interrogation strategies" as part of the Guantanamo and Abu Ghraib Behavioral Science Consultation Teams [26]. Several professionals have opposed this role based on ethical principles.

10.4 Diminishing the Harm

There are several ways in which evaluators can perform an objective evaluation and attempt to diminish the vulnerability of immigrants in forensic evaluations. Evaluators should be aware that each option has its own limitation and potential for bias.

Finding an evaluator of the same background is an obviously good option. These evaluators should be aware of their own limitations and may have to recuse themselves from a case if the limitations are such (e.g., strong countertransference) that they might affect their objectivity.

For an evaluator of different or similar ethnic background there are many other options. The evaluator should use a well-trained interpreter and become familiar with the evaluee's ethnic background. An evaluator has multiple sources to learn about the evaluee's ethnic background. One is to interview family members and other non-related members of the immigrant's community. The first group can be obviously biased. Other sources of information can come from other professionals, including anthropologists and cultural brokers. In the case of immigrants seeking asylum, official organizations from their country of origin might deny claims of torture or political persecution and in these cases collateral resources might include non-governmental agencies such as Amnesty International [8]. In other cases, sources of information can include the media, for example, the case of a Mexican American who was asking for relief under the UN Convention Against Torture. He said that if he were to return to his country he would not be able to afford his psychiatric medications and would end up in an Inpatient Unit in his country "under subhuman conditions" [27]. In his case, sources of information about the conditions in Mexican mental institutions included transcripts from an American television program called "20/20" and from a national public radio report [27].

Structured interviews and psychological tests are said to diminish bias in forensic evaluations. The problem is that "culturally adapted and validated testing instruments do not exist" [18] and a text translation does not validate the test [28,29]. For example, the Spanish version of the Composite International Diagnostic Interview may over-diagnose somatization in Hispanics [30].

10.4.1 The Transcultural Forensic Evaluation

A way to organize and systematically think about the information gathered is by using the transcultural forensic evaluation [12,31,32], which applies the elements of the *DSM-IV* clinical cultural formulation [33] to the forensic interview. The cultural formulation includes five sections; the transcultural forensic evaluation follows each in a forensic context:

1. **Cultural identity of the individual**. This section includes a narrative of the evaluee's ethnic background, "degree of involvement" with the culture of origin and the "host" culture, preferred language, and fluency in other languages. For example, a transcultural forensic evaluation of a Hispanic with Dissociative Identity Disorder showed that the different personalities had different degrees of involvement in the Hispanic versus the United States culture [32].

2. **Cultural explanations of the individual's illness and acts**. This section explains the "idioms of distress through which symptoms or the need for social support are communicated" [33]. It includes "preferences" of somatic over emotional symptoms, culture-bound syndromes, and views of origin and treatment of a given illness. For example, an immigrant might explain his or her symptoms as a result of witchcraft. The immigrant might then elaborate on how the witchcraft was done by a given person whom he or she felt compelled to attack to find relief [12].

3. **Cultural factors related to psychosocial environment and levels of functioning**. This section incorporates interpretations of social stressors, available social supports, and levels of functioning and disability. For example, a study showed how in a group of Central American immigrants "high levels of stress, increased perceptions of severity of disability" [34]. Although a single study does not determine a group's reality, it is important to consider whether such findings are true and refer to other studies and sources of information for clarification.

4. **Cultural elements of the relationship between the individual and the evaluator**. This section emphasizes the differences between each party which can influence the opinion (such as differences in body language, eye contact, and personal space). For example, some Arab women might not shake hands and might feel uncomfortable with direct eye contact [35].

5. **Overall cultural assessment for the opinion**. The section is a cultural formulation of the case.

Forensic evaluators can use many of the multiple options for gathering and organizing the information. The main goal is to diminish the bias to this vulnerable population by striving for objectivity. If there is any concern for bias, an evaluator can get further support by referring to professional ethical guidelines [36], consulting with ethical committees, consulting with colleagues who have more experience in transcultural evaluations.

10.5   Summary

Forensic psychiatrists are often called upon to evaluate immigrants in several different contexts. Most forensic evaluators will not be familiar with the ethnic background of the immigrant. This can result in biases arising from language barrier, misunderstanding about the immigrant's background, countertransference and transference. Immigrants are vulnerable to bias even when evaluated by someone of similar or same background. There are different ways of diminishing the bias; most of these are based on expanding the evaluator's knowledge on the immigrant's ethnic background. A way of expanding our knowledge as a professional community would be by investigating further the vulnerability and issues facing this population in the forensic context.

References

1. Migration Policy Institute (US) (2009) Frequently Requested Statistics on Immigrants and Immigration in the United States [Internet]. Migration Policy Institute (US), Washington, DC. Available from: http://www.migrationinformation.org/USfocus/display.cfm?ID=747 (accessed February 5, 2010).

2. United Nations, Department of Economic and Social Affairs, Statistics Division (1998) *Recommendations on Statistics of International Migration* [Internet], Statistical Papers Series M, No. 58, United Nations Publication, New York. Rev. 1. Available from: http://unstats.un.org/unsd/publication/SeriesM/SeriesM_58rev1E.pdf (accessed February 5, 2010).

3. United Nations, United Nations High Commissioner for Refugees (1997) *Convention and Protocol Relating to the Status of Refugees* [Internet]. UNHCR Media Relations and Public Information Service, Geneva. Available from: http://www.unhcr.org/protect/PROTECTION/3b66c2aa10.pdf (accessed February 5, 2010).

4. United States Department of Homeland Security, Office of Immigration Statistics (2009) *Annual Flow Report, Refugees and Asylees: 2008* [Internet]. Office of Immigration Statistics. Available from: http://www.dhs.gov/xlibrary/assets/statistics/publications/ois_rfa_fr_2008.pdf (accessed February 5, 2010).

5. United Nations, Department of Economic and Social Affairs, Statistics Division (2007) *Principles and Recommendations for Population and Housing Censuses* [Internet], Statistical papers Series M. No. 67, United Nations Publication, New York. Rev. 2. Available from: http://unstats.un.org/unsd/demographic/sources/census/docs/P&R_%20Rev2.pdf (accessed February 5, 2010).

6. Berk, M.L. and Schur, C.L. (2001) The effect of fear on access to care among undocumented Latino immigrants. *Journal of Immigrant Health*, **3**(3), 151–6.

7. Vega, W.A., Kolody, B., Aguilar-Gaxiola, S. *et al.* (1998) Lifetime prevalence of DSM-III-R psychiatric disorders among urban and rural Mexican Americans in California. *Archives of General Psychiatry*, **55**(9), 771–8.

8. Sarkar, S.P. (2009) Truth without consequence: reality and recall in refugees fleeing persecution. *Journal of the American Academy of Psychiatry and the Law*, **37**(1), 6–10.

9. Frumkin, B. and Friedland, J. (1995) Forensic evaluations in immigration cases: evolving issues. *Behavioral Science and the Law*, **13**(4), 477–89.

10. Vasquez, C. and Javier, R.A. (1991) The problem with interpreters: communicating with Spanish-speaking patients. *Hospital and Community Psychiatry*, **42**(2), 163–5.

11. Department of Justice (US), Executive Office for Immigration Review, Law Library and Immigration Research Center, Virtual Law Library (1982) *Matter of Exilus* [Internet]. Board of Immigration Appeals. 18 I&N Dec. 276. Available from: http://www.justice.gov/eoir/vll/intdec/vol18/2914.pdf (accessed February 6, 2010).

12. Silva, J.A., Leong, G.B., and Weinstock, R. (2003) Culture and ethnicity, in *Principles and Practice of Forensic Psychiatry*, 2nd edn (ed. R. Rosner), Arnold, London, pp. 631–42.

13. Hicks, J.W. (2004) Ethnicity, race, and forensic psychiatry: are we color-blind? *Journal of the American Academy of Psychiatry and the Law*, **32**(1), 21–33.

14. Migration Policy Institute (US) (2003) *America's Challenge: Domestic Security, Civil Liberties, and National Unity After September 11* [Internet]. Migration Policy Institute (US), Washington DC. Available from: http://www.migrationpolicy.org/pubs/Americas_Challenges.pdf (accessed February 6, 2010).

15. Liokis, M.G. and Herbert, P.B. (2005) Legal digest: competence to stand trial. *Journal of the American Academy of Psychiatry and the Law*, **33**(4), 554–5.

16. Evans, F.B. (2005) Trauma, torture, and transformation in the forensic assessor. *Journal of Personality Assessment*, **84**(1), 25–8; discussion 33–36.

17. Jong J. (2004) Public mental health and culture: Disasters as a challenge to western mental health care models, the self and PTSD, in *Broken Spirits: The Treatment of Traumatized Asylum Seekers, Refugees, War and Torture Victims*, 1st edn (eds. J.P. Wilson and B. Drodek), Brunner-Routledge, New York, pp. 159–78.

18. Kirmayer, L.J., Rousseau, C., and Lashley, M. (2007) The place of culture in forensic psychiatry. *Journal of the American Academy of Psychiatry and the Law*, **35**(1), 98–102.

19. Escobar, J.I. (1987) Cross-cultural aspects of the somatization trait. *Hospital and Community Psychiatry*, **38**(2), 174–80.

20. Chaleby, K.S. (1996) Issues in forensic psychiatry in Islamic jurisprudence. *Bulletin of the American Academy of Psychiatry and the Law*, **24**(1), 117–24.

21. Schlussel, D. (2009) Muslim Immigration Fraud Story of the Day [Internet]. Personal internet site. May 19. Available from: http://www.debbieschlussel.com/5203/muslim-immigration-fraud-story-of-the-day/ (accessed February 6, 2010).

22. Adetunji, B. (2009) My fellowship experience. *Newsletter American Academy of Psychiatry and the Law*, **34**(1), 16–17.

23. Sacks, V.L. (1996) An indefensible defense: on the misuse of culture in criminal law. *Arizona Journal of International and Comparative Law*, **13**, 523–50.

24. Rentel, A.D. (1993) A justification of the cultural defense as a partial excuse. *Southern California Review of Law and Women's Studies (RLAWS)*, **2**, 437–526.

25. Sams, J.P. (1986) The availability of the 'cultural defense' as an excuse for criminal behavior. *Georgia Journal of International and Comparative Law*, **16**, 335–54.

26. Janofsky, J.S. (2006) Lies and coercion: why psychiatrists should not participate in police and intelligence interrogations. *Journal of the American Academy of Psychiatry and the Law*, **34**(4), 472–8.

27. Torres, F.E. and Watson, C. (2009) Legal digest: a mentally ill alien's challenge to removal from the United States under the convention against torture. *Journal of the American Academy of Psychiatry and the Law*, **37**(3), 413–15.

28. Demsky, Y.I., Mittenberg, W., Quintar, B. *et al.* (1998) Bias in the use of standard American norms with Spanish translations of the Wechsler memory scale-revised. *Assessment*, **5**(2), 115–21.

29. López, S. and Romero, A. (1988) Assessing the intellectual functioning of Spanish-speaking adults: comparison of the EIWA and the WAIS. *Professional Psychology Research and Practice*, **19**(3), 263–70.

30. Villaseñor, Y. and Waitzkin, H. (1999) Limitations of a structured psychiatric diagnostic instrument in assessing somatization among Latino patients in primary care. *Medical Care*, **37**(7), 637–46.

31. Silva, J.A., Leong, G.B., Yamamoto, J. *et al.* (1997) A transcultural forensic psychiatric perspective of a mother who killed her children. *American Journal of Forensic Psychiatry*, **18**(3), 39–58.

32. Silva, J.A., Leong, G.B., and Derecho, D.V. (2000) Dissociative identity disorder: a transcultural forensic psychiatric analysis. *American Journal of Forensic Psychiatry*, **21**(3), 19–36.

33. American Psychiatric Association (2000) *Diagnostic and Statistical Manual of Mental Disorders, Text Revision*, 4th edn, Appendix I: Outline for Cultural Formulation and Glossary of Culture-Bound syndromes, American Psychiatric Publishing, Arlington.

34. Jarama, S.L., Reyst, H., Rodriguez, M. *et al.* (1998) Psychosocial adjustment among Central American immigrants with disabilities: an exploratory study. *Cultural Diversity and Mental Health*, **4**(2), 115–25.

35. Sparling, T. (2006) Caring for Fatima. *Journal of Clinical Oncology*, **24**(16), 2589–91.

36. American Academy of Psychiatry and the Law (US) (2005) *American Academy of Psychiatry and the Law Ethics Guidelines for the Practice of Forensic Psychiatry*. Adopted May. Available from: http://www.aapl.org/ethics.htm (accessed February 6, 2010).

11 Prisoners and Death Row Inmates

Robert L. Sadoff

University of Pennsylvania School of Medicine, Philadelphia, USA

11.1 Introduction

Correctional psychiatry is included in forensic psychiatry and is taught as an essential element in accredited training programs in forensic psychiatry. The treatment of individuals in prison has also been referred to as forensic psychotherapy. The psychiatrist working within the prison system, treating the mentally ill, faces a number of ethical issues. A conflict may occur between a secure environment and a therapeutic environment; when the two conflict in the prison system, security trumps therapy. However, psychiatrists have made great inroads in effecting changes within our correctional system that provide for therapy for those in need.

There are special housing units for protective custody of those who are vulnerable, such as those who have been convicted of child sexual crimes, racial crimes, political crimes, and terrorist crimes. There are also special units for those inmates who are psychotic, or become psychotic, within the prison system. There are special units for passive, weak, effeminate-appearing males who may become victims of sexual assault. Provisions have also been made to transfer the extremely mentally ill to correctional hospital facilities where they will receive treatment in a safe and therapeutic environment.

However, there are individuals who have been committed to prison who have been taking particular medications for mental illness, which are not allowed in the prison. Substitutes often have to be made that may not be appropriate or as helpful to the inmate. Psychiatrists working within the prison system who are limited in the type and quality of medication available have to make creative judgments about the treatment of their patients within the system. A number of facilities are short-handed and do not have sufficient medical coverage for adequate treatment.

Ethical Issues in Forensic Psychiatry: Minimizing Harm by Robert L. Sadoff
© 2011 John Wiley & Sons, Ltd

Occasionally, inmates have to wait a fairly long time in order to be seen and given proper treatment. Sometimes, they have to be transferred to another facility for treatment of their particular mental illness. Inmates have complained that they do not get adequate treatment, and have difficulty getting appointments with medical personnel. Other facilities are well staffed, and patients obtain adequate and sufficient treatment.

It is my contention that mentally ill, mentally retarded, and other individuals within the prison system are a vulnerable population that need to be treated appropriately and within the ethical guidelines of AAPL, AMA, and APA.

11.2   The Role of Mental Health Professionals in Prisons

Metzner and Dvoskin [1] discuss the role of the mental health professional within the correctional setting. They begin with the seriously mentally ill inmates in supermax prisons, and talk about the rapidly escalating rate of incarceration in the United States that has been associated with an increasing number of imprisoned individuals who suffer from mental illness.

They note that as many as 20% of inmates in jail and prison are in need of psychiatric care for serious mental illness. The US Bureau of Justice statistics estimate 283 800 mentally ill offenders were incarcerated in US prisons and jails at midyear 1998 [1]. The authors focus on several evolving issues in correctional mental health care that are especially controversial and often inadequately addressed within correctional facilities. For example, they discuss the issue of segregation and isolation and whether isolation is mentally harmful to the inmates. They note that there are several different statuses that can result from segregation. Disciplinary segregation, typically ordered as punishment for an institutional infraction, is often of short duration. In contrast, administrative segregation is typically imposed based on what the inmate might do. That is, administrative segregation is prospective in nature and designed to protect other inmates from a danger believed to be posed by the inmate.

The authors present three situations that result in segregation status which require different institutional responses.

1. First, inmates who, either because they are unable or unwilling, fail to abide by institutional rules, thereby creating a danger to institutional order, security, or the safety of staff and inmates.
2. The second type of segregation inmate is one who knows well how to negotiate a correctional environment, but whose wish for power and money leads him or her to join and even lead prison gangs in the perpetration of organized crime within the prison. These inmates are leaders or "shot callers" of prison gangs and are believed to pose such an extreme danger to other prisoners that they can never return to general population.
3. In some states, inmates find their way into long-term segregation because their mental and intellectual limitations prevent them from following orders and successfully following prison rules. They state: "No one should ever be

placed in long-term segregation because of their serious mental disability or its symptoms" [1].

Further, the authors note,

There is general consensus among clinicians that placement of inmates with serious mental illnesses in long-term segregated settings is contraindicated because many of these inmates' psychiatric conditions will clinically deteriorate or not improve. In other words, many inmates with serious mental illnesses are harmed when placed in a supermax setting, especially if they are not given access to necessary psychological and psychiatric care. In addition to potential litigation, this is one of the main reasons that many states (e.g., Ohio, California, Illinois, and Wisconsin) exclude inmates with serious mental illnesses from admission to supermax facilities [1].

The authors conclude: "No one should be housed in segregation while they are acutely psychotic, suicidal, or otherwise in the midst of a psychiatric crisis. The exceptions would be the most extraordinary and dangerous circumstances." The authors go on to describe more appropriate treatment recommendations for this population, which would reduce the harm to these vulnerable individuals [1].

11.3 Death Penalty Issues

Appelbaum [2] has expressed his concern about the ethical conflict of the psychiatrist working in a prison that houses death row inmates. The death row inmate who becomes severely psychotic and requires psychiatric treatment with medication may pose an ethical challenge for the treating psychiatrist. Is it ethical for the psychiatrist to treat such individuals in order to make them competent so that they may be executed by the state? Many psychiatrists would refuse to work in such an environment in order to avoid facing that ethical dilemma.

Other psychiatrists would work in the institution and justify their treatment of the mentally ill inmate on death row in order to alleviate the pain and suffering of the acutely psychotic individual and to, hopefully, help him or her become competent in order to perhaps find, with their attorney, that one "scintilla of evidence" that would exonerate them, or at least remove them from death row.

Leong *et al.* [3] found, from a survey of board certified forensic psychiatrists in the United States, that most respondents supported a role, in at least some cases, for a forensic evaluation of prisoners accused of capital crimes. Respondents were divided on whether or not psychiatrists should treat incompetent death row prisoners if restoration of competence would result in execution. Attitudes about the ethical acceptability of capital punishment were associated with views about the psychiatrist's role, but were not determinative in every case.

The AMA has made it very clear that it is unethical for physicians to participate in death penalty cases [4]. By that, they meant when execution was done by lethal injection rather than by firing squad, hanging, or electrocution, that the physician should not be the one to inject the lethal material into the inmate's body, causing his or her death. Forensic psychiatrists were challenged by the AMA mandate about participating in capital cases, or death penalty cases. They wondered whether they could testify for the prosecution about mitigating or aggravating circumstances in such cases. Initially, a number of psychiatrists refused to participate for the prosecution inasmuch as their testimony could lead to the death of the defendant if found guilty. However, a number of psychiatrists were comfortable working for the defense in finding mitigating factors that could possibly spare the life of the defendant mandating a life sentence rather than the death penalty. It became a serious ethical question for forensic psychiatrists requested by the prosecution to rebut the testimony of those defense psychiatrists who found significant mitigating evidence that would outweigh the aggravating factors and spare the life of the defendant.

Another major dilemma occurred for forensic psychiatrists who were asked by judges to evaluate the competency of death row inmates to stop their appeals. All capital cases that result in a death penalty verdict are automatically appealed and assessed by the higher court. Some cases go to the Supreme Court several times before final adjudication and the death sentence is carried out. Sometimes these cases take years to prepare, and the death row inmate deteriorates in their environment, which is quite restrictive, over several years or even decades.

Occasionally, a death row inmate will decide not to pursue his or her appeals and will tell their attorneys that they are not going to appeal any further and want to be put to death. The attorneys fighting for their life will question their competency to stop their appeals, and will retain forensic mental health experts to assess the competency of the inmate to pursue their appeals. In these cases, we can have another "battle of the experts," as occurred in the case of Heidnick [5], in which four psychiatrists—two for the prosecution and two for the defense—interviewed Gary Heidnick at the same time for several hours in front of attorneys and others to determine whether he was competent to stop his appeals. There was a mixed opinion divided between the two prosecution psychiatrists and the two for the defense. The judge found that Heidnick was competent to stop his appeals, and he was subsequently executed.

George Banks [6] was a seriously mentally ill individual when he killed 13 people in one night, including several of his own children. Even though he was mentally ill, he was determined to be not legally insane and was convicted of the 13 murders and given the death penalty.

Banks had been deteriorating on death row for 22 years when his competency to be executed was challenged by his appellate attorneys. It was clear that he had deteriorated to such a point that he could no longer understand the nature and consequences of his legal situation and could not understand why he was being put to death. He was seen by several psychiatrists for the defense and for the prosecution, and testimony was given over a period of time. The judge determined that he was incompetent to be executed, and he was returned to his prison cell.

Here is an example of a very vulnerable individual put into the system, and treatment was unsuccessful. Because he was on death row, his movements were limited, and his treatment was restricted. He was determined to be unfit or incompetent to be executed and was returned to the prison system. However, because the death sentence was commuted, and if the appeals by the prosecution for a new hearing are not successful, he will not return to death row and, hopefully, will be able to obtain necessary treatment within the system that may not have been available to him while he was on death row.

Kermani and Kantor [7] present the landmark Supreme Court cases on death penalty and their ethical implications for forensic psychiatrists. The authors note that the US Supreme Court had made a number of recent rulings in regard to the death penalty that will likely have the effect of increasing the use of expert psychiatric testimony during the trial and sentencing process in capital cases. They also note that any such changes are bound to increase the number of ethical dilemmas faced by psychiatrists involved in such work. They note the rulings that affect psychiatry include:

1. The Eighth Amendment forbids the execution of persons who are mentally incompetent in regard to their ability to appreciate the reasons for punishment.
2. A mentally ill prisoner may be forcibly given neuroleptics if he or she presents a danger to themselves or others.
3. Forced medication may not be used during the trial and sentencing phase if it has the potential to change the defendant's demeanor significantly enough to affect his or her defense.
4. Aggravating psychological factors affecting a convictee may be balanced against mitigating factors in considering whether death sentence should be imposed.
5. The psychosocial impact of the crime upon the victim's family may be presented during the sentencing phase as factors relevant to sentencing.
6. Adolescents and retarded individuals are not immune from the death penalty simply by virtue of their age or level of intelligence. (Later cases did exclude the mentally retarded (Penry) [8] and juveniles (Atkins) [9] from the death penalty.)

The two landmark cases utilized are *Perry v. Louisiana* [10] and *Riggins v. Nevada* [11]. In Perry, the issue is whether the state may forcibly treat an incompetent inmate with antipsychotic drugs in order to make him competent for execution. In Riggins, the issue is whether the state may forcibly medicate a mentally ill defendant in order to restore his competency to stand trial for charges in which a guilty verdict might result in his execution. The authors also cite *Washington v. Harper* [12], which was a precedent case and indicates that states can forcibly medicate an incompetent prisoner, but first the state must establish that

1. the incompetent prisoner is dangerous to him- or herself or others or is seriously disruptive to the functioning of the penal institution, and
2. that the treatment is in the inmate's medical interest.

The US Supreme Court found that persons with mental retardation were not automatically precluded for being executed upon conviction for a capital crime [8]. In cases of mental retardation, the jury must weigh the defendant's mental status as indicative of a possibility that there may have been related circumstances that may mitigate against capital punishment. Relevant mitigating factors could include poor moral reasoning and lack of ability to understand basic relationships between actions and their consequences.

The authors note, "The ethical codes of the APA and AMA in their present forms condemn physicians who forcibly medicate an inmate for the purposes of grooming him for execution" [4]. The same code of ethics also dictates that minors and individuals with retardation should not be punished by the death sentence. The authors note that the Supreme Court rulings created new ethical dilemmas for psychiatry. "The moral principle of non maleficence and beneficence appears inconsistent both with some of the interests of the justice system and with the desires of a society which would prefer to bring violators to quick and final punishment" [7].

The authors conclude with these comments to our colleagues:

> *Psychiatrists who intend to participate in the implementation of justice, have an obligation to weigh several factors, including their own beliefs about the institution of punishment, their moral obligations as physicians, their civic duties as citizens, and their beliefs about a patient defendant's rights in regard to consent for medical care. Decisions whether or not to participate in such processes should be based on well considered personal principles and moral values, rather than on blind obedience to professional codes of ethics or institutional job descriptions [7].*

Weinstock [13] notes that as a result of recent decisions by the US Supreme Court and the California Supreme Court, "Therapists now have been placed in a position in which they can be forced to testify in death penalty cases for the only purposes of achieving a conviction and death penalty verdict." Further, he notes, "In California, therapists can now be forced to testify against their own patients in capital cases even if the patient does not tender his mental state as an issue, despite the presence of a psychotherapist patient privilege in the state for criminal matters" [13].

Edersheim and Beck [14] review the literature and note that the presence or absence of expert testimony could play a critical role in jury sentencing decisions. They indicate,

> *All states now have a bifurcated trial process for capital defendants. The first phase of the trial is the innocence or guilt phase, and if the defendant is found guilty, the trial proceeds to the penalty or sentencing phase. During the penalty phase, the jury hears so-called 'aggravation' testimony from the prosecution and 'mitigation' testimony from the defense which is typically favorable evidence regarding the defendant's history, character, and mental condition [14].*

The authors also cite the case of *Strickland v. Washington* [15], in which the Supreme Court imposes a low standard of competence for criminal attorneys regarding the evaluation of claims of ineffective assistance of counsel. The authors note that psychiatrists may be called to testify that the defense attorney at trial failed to call a mental health professional to alert the jury to the specific illnesses or problems, or even history of the defendant. The appellate lawyer would argue that had the jury heard this information, they might have concluded differently on the death penalty.

Beck discusses his experience with assessing individuals charged with capital crimes [16]. He notes the mental retardation of one, which would excuse him from being executed because of the Supreme Court decision in Penry that prohibits executing the mentally retarded. Clearly, the mentally retarded are a vulnerable group in the judicial system as are those charged with capital offenses. The psychiatrist in death row cases is utilized primarily to gather information and data for mitigation in order to avoid the death penalty. Psychiatrists for the prosecution may find there is no mitigating circumstance and do not comment on the aggravating factors that are not psychiatric.

Beck presents three cases, and notes that two of the cases directly illustrate the value of psychiatric input to defense in cases of capital murder. "Paradoxically, the psychiatric contribution in one case was to portray the defendant as mentally disordered, while in the other it was to portray him as without any disorder. This latter case illustrates more forcibly than any argument that the psychiatrist best serves his or her client by accurate observation and truthful reporting, rather than by slanting or distorting findings or testimony." Beck concludes, "Psychiatric participation serves not only the individual defendant, but the more abstract value of equal justice under law" [16].

With regard to the concept of "First, do no harm," the authors of an article in *Psychiatric News*, 1990 [17], state that "Do no harm is ambiguous in the context of correctional work." They state,

> *It is not clear why adherence to the 'Do no harm' principle should not enjoin physicians from participating in any process that helps enable any sort of punishment for patients, capital or not. Presumably, any punishment meted out to a convicted criminal could be construed as harm to the person punished. The same objection may be presented to those who would be willing to participate in making condemned convictees competent if they could be assured that the prisoner's punishment by execution would be commuted to life imprisonment [17].*

In linking those comments to correctional psychiatry and the death penalty, the authors also argue that "restoring a person by treating him is not in keeping with putting him in a state of mental well being, especially if he is going to be executed." They argue that psychiatrists "have a duty of beneficence and that being beneficent in acting in the patient's best interest can no longer be seen simply as providing 'happiness for the patient.' In principle, that goal of psychiatry to restore autonomy may be quite consistent with helping to make a person competent to be executed" [17].

Finally, the authors cite other objections to treating a person in order to make him or her competent to be executed and note the moral balance against the psychiatrist taking part in tacit or causal factors leading to execution are the following:

- if the psychiatrist believes that the institution of capital punishment is morally wrong, whether or not its implementation requires the help of psychiatrists;

- if the goal of the "treatment" of the individual prisoner is specifically to enable execution;
- if the task is being undertaken contrary to the convicted's wishes.

The authors note, "Under the doctrine of beneficence, autonomy is important and the person's wishes need to be considered" [17].

In cases of juveniles or the mentally retarded, psychiatrists can make a difference in testifying about the maturity of the juvenile or minor, and the mental ability and competence of the mentally retarded. The case of *Thompson v. Oklahoma* [18] barred execution of inmates under the age of 16 at the time of their offense.

In the case of mental retardation, the holding case is *Penry v. Lynaugh* [8], where Penry had an IQ between 50 and 63, indicative of mild to moderate mental retardation. He was found competent to stand trial. In the sentencing procedure, the jury, in accordance with state law, confirmed that the murder was deliberate and that there was probability that Penry would commit further violent crimes. In that jurisdiction, being a continuing threat to society meant that he must be sentenced to death. When the case came before the US Supreme Court, the justices were confronted with two questions:

- whether Penry's rights were violated because the jury was not adequately instructed to take all of the mitigating circumstances, including mental retardation, into consideration;
- secondly, whether it would be cruel and unusual punishment under the Eighth Amendment to execute a person with mental retardation with Penry's reasoning ability.

In all death penalty cases, aggravating and mitigating factors are significant, and the psychiatrist becomes involved in mitigating factors, not the aggravating ones. However, the prosecution may call an expert psychiatrist to rebut the existence of mitigating factors presented by the defense expert.

In summary, these are the vulnerable people within the correctional system that require sensitivity and special handling by the forensic mental health expert so that we do not aggravate their conditions and do further harm especially to those facing the death penalty. Here, we have another opportunity to minimize the harm that is inherent in the system if we proceed with sensitivity, with caution, and with concern for the welfare of the vulnerable individual within the judicial and correctional system.

References

1. Metzner, J. and Dvoskin, J. (2006) An overview of correctional psychiatry. *Psychiatric Clinics of North America*, **29**(3), 761–72.
2. Appelbaum, P.S. (1997) A theory of ethics for forensic psychiatry. *Journal of the American Academy of Psychiatry and the Law*, **25**, 233–47.
3. Leong, G.B., Silva, J.A., Weinstock, R., and Ganzini, L. (2000) Survey of forensic psychiatrists on evaluation and treatment of prisoners on death row. *Journal of the American Academy of Psychiatry and the Law*, **28**, 427–32.

4. American Psychiatric Association (2008) *The Principles of Medical Ethics With Annotations Especially Applicable to Psychiatry*, Washington, DC.

5. *Commonwealth v. Heidnik*, 526 Pa. 458, 587 A.2d 687, (1991).

6. *Beard v. Banks*, 542 US 406, 124, S.Ct. 2504, 159L Ed. 2d 494 (2004).

7. Kermani, E.J. and Kantor, J.E. (1994) Psychiatry and the death penalty: the landmark supreme court cases and their ethical implications for the profession. *Bulletin of the American Academy of Psychiatry and the Law*, **22**, 95–108.

8. *Penry v. Lynaugh*, 492 US 302 (1989).

9. *Atkins v. Virginia*, 536 US 304, (2002).

10. *Perry v. Louisiana*, 498 US 38, (1990).

11. *Riggins v. Nevada*, 504 US 127, (1992).

12. *Washington v. Harper*, 494 US 210, (1990).

13. Weinstock, R. (1994) Utilizing therapists to obtain death penalty verdicts. *Bulletin of the American Academy of Psychiatry and the Law*, **22**, 39–52.

14. Edersheim, J.G. and Beck, J.C. (2005) Commentary: expert testimony as a potential asset in defense of capital sentencing cases. *Journal of the American Academy of Psychiatry and the Law*, **33**, 519–22.

15. *Strickland v. Washington*, 466 US 668, (1984).

16. Beck, J.C. (1993) The role of psychiatry and death penalty defense. *Bulletin of the American Academy of Psychiatry and the Law*, **21**, 453–63.

17. (1990) Death row inmates shouldn't be made to become competent. *American Psychiatric News*, **25**(15), 2.

18. *Thompson v. Oklahoma*, 487 US 815, (1988).

12 Forensic Psychiatric Experts: Risks and Liability

Robert L. Sadoff

University of Pennsylvania School of Medicine, Philadelphia, USA

12.1 Introduction

In previous chapters, we have presented the potential harm that could occur to the forensic mental health expert during the psychiatric examination, as a result of report writing and during testimony in court. This chapter will serve to elaborate on the various dangers that may befall the mental health expert in conducting forensic psychiatric assessments. The dangers may occur as a result of the type of individual examined; for example, a borderline female who accuses the examiner of boundary crossings or violations. Lawsuits may occur to the forensic expert either as a result of incomplete examination, inappropriate modification of his or her report, and/or exaggeration or improper comments during testimony. There are also a number of conflicts that may face the forensic expert that could cause emotional harm.

With respect to medical malpractice liability, Weinstock and Garrick [1] point out that forensic psychiatrists are not as vulnerable to liability as general psychiatrists. The absence of a physician-patient relationship and traditional immunity are all protective against malpractice actions. Although the absence of a doctor-patient relationship removes the essential element of malpractice, other types of liability such as defamation and ordinary negligence are possible. The authors indicate that forensic psychiatrists are immune if there is no doctor-patient relationship, but if they are sued for other reasons, they may not be covered by their malpractice insurance.

Ethical Issues in Forensic Psychiatry: Minimizing Harm   by Robert L. Sadoff
© 2011 John Wiley & Sons, Ltd

12.2   Malpractice Considerations

In perhaps the most comprehensive study of liability for psychiatric experts, Binder [2] reviewed the medical and legal literature about expert witness immunity. She found that the traditional concepts of expert witness immunity reveal how a variety of factors have led to the erosion of this immunity. These factors include the proliferation of experts, the inadequacy of traditional safeguards of potential prosecution for perjury in cross-examination, the growth of attorney malpractice, the lack of protection of the injured party from unscrupulous witnesses, and the ineffectiveness of *Daubert v. Merrell Dow Pharmaceuticals* [3]. Examples are given to show how expert witnesses are being held accountable by professional associations and state medical boards and through tort liability. She concludes by providing risk management strategies and guidelines for psychiatrists who are considering engaging in forensic work.

Binder notes the witness immunity doctrine originated hundreds of years ago in English common law for broad public policy reasons. The intent of witness immunity has been to encourage open and honest testimony without fear of a subsequent lawsuit related to the testimony. Courts have upheld the immunity doctrine and in the 1980s there were two cases in the US Supreme Court. One is *Briscoe v. LaHue* (1983) [4], and the other is *Mitchell v. Forsyth* (1985) [5].

Binder presents precedent-setting cases: one is New Jersey Supreme Court, *Levine v. Wiss & Co.* [6] against an accountant; another is *Pettus v. Cole et al.* [7] a claim of negligence against an accounting firm, and a third, Missouri Supreme Court, *Murphy v. A.A. Matthews* [8]. The Missouri Supreme Court held, in a case against engineers, that witness immunity does not bar lawsuits against professional expert witnesses for alleged negligence in reaching opinions.

Binder presents two unpublished cases against psychiatrists. In one case, in performing a fitness-for-duty evaluation of an employee, a psychiatrist diagnosed the employee as having a paranoid personality disorder and the employee was suspended. The employee brought a lawsuit against the psychiatrist, retained an expert witness who discredited the basis of the diagnosis by saying that the paranoid personality was inaccurate and that the thoughts of conspiracy by the employee were related to cultural ideas rather than to a psychiatric diagnosis. The employee represented himself, but the psychiatrist had to go out and hire his own attorney and experts to determine whether or not the diagnosis of paranoid personality was reasonable. The causative actions were dismissed after several years of aggravation and stress for the psychiatrist/defendant.

In a second case, a psychiatrist was asked to evaluate a disability claim brought by a 45-year-old man with recurrent depression. She interviewed the man, wrote a report stating that his complaints were consistent with a major depressive disorder and supported his claim of disability. Subsequent to the writing of the report, the man's insurance company showed the psychiatrist a surveillance videotape made of this businessman. The videotape showed that after leaving the psychiatrist's office, the man was laughing and conversing with an acquaintance as he went shopping in the neighborhood. This was in contrast with what the man had reported to the psychiatrist. He told the psychiatrist he was barely able to move and could not engage in pleasurable activities. On the basis of this brief surveillance videotape, the psychiatrist wrote a supplemental report in which she stated that she was changing her diagnosis to malingering. As a result of this supplemental report, the man's disability claim was denied. He brought a lawsuit against the evaluating psychiatrist, and three causes of action were set forth: defamation, intentional infliction of emotional distress, and conspiracy. The psychiatrist's attorney requested a consultation to determine whether the psychiatrist's diagnosis of malingering was reached within the standards of practice for forensic psychiatrists. The attorney tried to have the defamation cause of action dismissed on the basis of the fact that psychiatrists have a qualified privilege related to their opinions; however, the court allowed the cause of action to proceed in its demurrer. The case is currently in litigation.

12.3 Helpful Recommendations

Binder gives guidelines for psychiatric expert witnesses to keep out of trouble. She says, "Psychiatrists should have training regarding the conduct of forensic evaluations before undertaking such work. They should also be aware of the ethical codes related to forensic work, such as the guidelines of the American Academy of Psychiatry and the Law (AAPL). Psychiatrists need to be certain they have the time to meet court deadlines and requirements" [9]. She gives seven different recommendations, as follows:

- Not specifying likely results or opinion and/or advertising how your services will achieve that result.
- Arranging fees and expenses, including retainers, at the outset of consultation.
- Maintaining strict records, including audiotaping or videotaping interviews when appropriate.
- Keeping the attorney informed of your opinion as it develops.
- Not overstating your opinions.
- Not taking cases beyond your ability and expertise.
- Preserving the attorney's and client's confidence as specified in the legal proceedings in which you are involved.

She concludes that psychiatrists should be certain they have malpractice coverage that will support their defense in the event they are sued in reference to forensic work.

Binder's recommendations are excellent and should be adhered to by all forensic psychiatrists in order to avoid getting into further difficulty. Specifically, fees should always be agreed upon at the outset, and often in writing, so there is no controversy or confusion or disagreement. Accurate records are very important to maintain in order to avoid conflict and disputes; audiotape or videotape may be helpful, or even necessary. Not overstating one's opinion is extremely important, especially when writing reports or discussing the matter with attorneys or the subjects themselves, and especially when testifying in court. One should be an advocate for one's opinions, but should not be the adversary in the case. These cases are adversarial in nature, but we need not argue the attorney's case.

Another extremely important concern raised by Binder is not accepting cases that go beyond our ability or expertise. I have alluded to cases that I would refuse on the basis of bias, but there are also cases that one should not accept on the basis of lack of experience, training, or competence. For example, I would not take a case involving a young girl involved in an accident because one would need to have a child or adolescent psychiatrist who has training in forensic work and in issues of growth and development. I would also refer, to a female forensic psychiatrist, cases involving women who have been sexually or violently abused by men. The elderly may be involved in legal matters that require the experience and training of a geriatric psychiatrist who also has forensic training.

The psychiatrist who testifies in court may do so either as a fact witness if he or she is the therapist, or as an expert witness if he or she is involved in the forensic assessment. There is liability for fact witnesses because of the well-established physician-patient relationship. For expert witness liability, the exposure may fall into any of three categories: malpractice lawsuits, discipline by the licensing board, and peer review and discipline by professional organizations. The expert may also be named in the National Practitioner Data Bank.

State medical boards may have special requirements for out-of-state witnesses, including licensure in the state for forensic activity [10]. (It should be noted that the AMA has deemed expert medical testimony as the practice of medicine.)[1] If such requirements are not followed, the out-of-state expert could be accused of practicing medicine without a license, and that could result in civil and/or criminal penalties as well as possibly voiding his/her malpractice insurance coverage.[2] The AMA has recommended that temporary licenses be required for out-of-state forensic examinations and testimony.[3] The AMA has also recommended that all expert witnesses be subject to peer review [11]. The AMA has ethical guidelines for experience in the area in which the individual testifies and limits testimony to that sphere of medical expertise [12].

All of this goes to the issue of minimizing harm, not only to the examinee, but also to the professional. Having the most thorough expertise and training will not only provide the best service to the individual and to his or her attorney, but also the best protection to our profession and to ourselves.

12.4 Danger of Violence to Forensic Experts

A recent study by Leavitt and others [13] has undertaken to add to the body of knowledge regarding the nature and frequency of assaults on mental health professionals in the context of their forensic practice as distinct from the general clinical practice. They mailed a four-page questionnaire to all individuals who had ever been admitted to the DFP (Designated Forensic Professional Credential

---

[1] AMA No. H265.993.
[2] Penalties vary depending on the jurisdiction.
[3] AMA No. H265.992.

Program), and a total of 190 were surveyed. One hundred and three (54%) were completed and returned. The respondents were 42% female and 57% male, a much higher percentage of psychologists (85%) than psychiatrists (15%). About half of the sample reported they had been the subject of at least one overt act of physical aggression; 29% of the respondents reported at least one such incident occurred in the course of their forensic work, and an equal percentage reported experiencing at least one incident in their general non-forensic practice. Most of them fell in the category of assault toward self without a weapon. None of the assaults with weapons included a gun or knife, but most often involved thrown objects: for example, comb, cup, cup of coffee, bottle of urine, and one involved the use of a sharpened toothbrush. There were no forced sexual assaults or acts. Most of the sexual assaults consisted of the evaluee's exposing himself, and the next largest category was incidents of inappropriate touching. There was minor property damage. One incident of aggression toward family involved slashing the tires of the evaluator's family car when it was parked at home.

The authors then surveyed the most distressing incident (MDI). Seventy-eight of the 103, or 76% chose to report the MDI they had encountered in the course of their forensic work. These are the examples: the father of a juvenile who was evaluated threatened the judge, the District Attorney, the psychiatrist, and his family. There were inappropriate, unwarranted threats from a judge, requiring another judge to calm him down; later, the judge apologized. Also, there were episodic stalking, unwelcome phone calls, letters, and packages showing up at a colleague's home. In a particular case, while a psychologist was testifying at a competence to stand trial hearing, the defendant's attorney suddenly approached, began yelling at the psychologist about his opinion. The judge admonished him, and he backed off. At the conclusion of the hearing the lawyer again came toward the psychologist in the courtroom, irate about his opinion. In another case, a sex offender defendant with a diagnosis of schizophrenia, began masturbating under the table. In another case, false complaints were filed against the psychiatrist with the Licensing Board in his state.

Thus, the present study reveals that 85% of the respondents had been harassed or intimidated, 65% had been threatened, and nearly 50% had been subjected to acts of actual physical aggression at least once during the course of their professional careers. There was no more overall aggression in respondents' forensic practice than in their non-forensic practice. Respondents who were victims of aggressive incidents did not differ by gender in any of the three categories of aggression. Thus, there was no more risk in the forensic than in the non-forensic context.

The study further found that forensic clinicians' concerns about their safety may be somewhat misplaced. For many mental health professionals, it is the fear of serious injury or death that looms large. In reality, it appears more likely that they will have to confront multiple aggressive incidents that leave no physical scars.

With respect to the MDI, "of the 78 respondents who chose to describe an incident, only three reported suffering any physical injury (two scratches, one injury scarring the face), and none were confronted with weapons such as guns or knives. Yet 27, or 35% of individuals required from several hours to several months to recover emotionally from the event." The authors conclude, "Attention to the emotional sequelae of what may seem to be the minor aggressive incidents is warranted. This should be highlighted in training programs to help clinicians to more realistically anticipate, assess, and care for their own emotional responses to these events. On an institutional level, there may be a need to develop a culture in which strong emotional reactions to aggressive incidents are legitimized, normalized, and respected" [13].

To our knowledge, there has been only one study specifically addressing the assaults on forensic evaluators, and that was when Miller [14] mailed a questionnaire to all 850 members of AAPL inquiring about their experience with verbal harassment or verbal threats or actions "in connection with their involvement as expert witnesses in forensic cases." He found a 48% response rate and that 42% of the sample had been harassed in some way: 17% had received threats of physical harm; 13% had received threats of non-violent injury; and 12% had received both types of threats. Three percent of the responders had actually been physically attacked, but no serious injuries were reported. In Miller's study, more than half of the reported assaults were committed by "attorneys, relatives, or others who were clearly not the ones being evaluated" [15].

Kroll and Mackenzie [16] state, "In an era of rapid discharge in community treatment, psychiatrists must assess with insufficient information, their patient's potential for committing a violent act outside of the hospital every time they authorize a pass or a discharge." The authors discuss a risk management approach to decision making that consists of three components: risk assessment, risk evaluation, and risk reduction. They also provide a decision table that clinicians can use to identify "factors that suggest a high risk of violence in a patient, a patient's current status, history, and treatment response."

This paper is cited in order to demonstrate the risk to psychiatrists in discharging patients from involuntary commitment to hospitals where they had been sent because of previous violent behavior. It is extremely important for the psychiatrist discharging such patients to consider risk assessments so as to avoid harm to the patients, to others in the community, or to the psychiatrists. If the patient goes on to harm someone after discharge, the psychiatrist ordering the discharge may be subject to a civil lawsuit for premature release that led to harm to others. However, the authors point out that legal judgments provide fairly good assurance that reasonable decisions supported by good records and clear communications will offer protection against liability for patients' assaults and suicides outside of the hospital. Further they note, "Nevertheless, there are compelling reasons for us continually to reassess and improve our clinical and decision-making procedures. These reasons include the safety of the patients and the public in general, as well as our professional need for greater competence" [16].

These considerations are important not only to protect society and the individual, but also to prevent further malpractice charges against treating psychiatrists. Petrilla and Sadoff [17] wrote on minimizing the risk of such discharge by communicating with the families of those who are being discharged to limit potential risk of violence.

12.5   Emotional Harm to Experts

There is another danger of harm to the expert, and that is the emotional toll that it takes on the mental health professional. This is an area that is never discussed and yet has great impact on mental health practitioners. Psychiatrists are trained to be helping individuals, and most prefer to maintain that posture. When they enter the forensic arena, however, there are differences and changes that are very uncomfortable for a number of psychiatrists.

I have had the opportunity of training a number of residents and postgraduate psychiatrists in forensic psychiatry at the University of Pennsylvania. I have experienced psychiatrists wishing to become involved in forensic cases and then becoming uncomfortable when actually having to testify against a plaintiff in a civil case or against a defendant in a criminal case.

One example is a female psychiatrist who was asked to examine a teacher who had been charged with boundary violations with one of his female students. She was a teenager under the age of consent who fell in love with her young gym teacher, and there was a sexual contact that led to his arrest and being fired from his job. The psychiatrist was asked to examine him with respect to his mental stability to return to a reasonable job that did not involve youngsters who may be potential victims of future boundary violations. She found that he had serious problems that prevented him from taking good jobs, despite the fact that youngsters would not be involved. She felt bad about testifying against him to keep him from working and had recriminations and self-doubts about how to write the report and how to approach the case in court.

Serving as a mentor in forensic cases can be very satisfying, but also challenging, especially when one encounters psychiatrists who have reasonable ethical concerns. She felt bad about what she was going to have to do that negatively affected this individual. She had been used to treating people, helping them in a therapeutic context, and this was brand new for her. My job was to help reassure her that if he had serious problems and had already acted on them to the detriment of one young teenager, it is likely that if he were placed in a position of responsibility that he could abuse his trust in the future and that others would be negatively impacted. To prevent harm to the community, she was encouraged to proceed even though her testimony would be harmful to him and his ability to get a job in his particular area.

A number of psychiatrists stay out of the forensic field because they do not wish to harm others, and when they find themselves in a position where they have to testify and cause harm, they have self-doubt and often have difficulty sleeping and require either therapy or reassurance that they are doing what is appropriate and ethical.

I have also had the experience of taking a group of young psychiatrists into a county prison to expose them to the type of treatment that people get even in the best of jails. On at least three occasions, individual psychiatrists were not able to go into the prison behind the clanging of the bars locking them in, because of claustrophobic or other uncomfortable fears.

Gutheil [18] has written about the impact on various psychiatrists when uncomfortable questions are asked on cross-examination, especially personal questions about divorce, about fees, about total income, or other matters which are usually kept personal and private, but not when a forensic case is in open court.

In a particular case of malpractice against a forensic psychiatrist, *Harris v. Kreutzer* [19], Ms. Harris contended that Dr. Kreutzer owed a duty to her to exercise reasonable and ordinary care and to avoid causing her harm in the conduct of his forensic examination. She argued that Dr. Kreutzer breached his duty by not complying with the applicable standard of care for his profession, and claimed that he was "deliberately abusive" and acted "with disregard for the consequences of his conduct," which led her mental and physical health to drastically deteriorate. She noted specific examples of such conduct, alleging Dr. Kreutzer "verbally abused her, raised his voice to her, caused her to break down in tears in his office, stating she was 'putting on a show' and accused her of being a faker and malingerer." She also contended that Dr. Kreutzer had prior knowledge of her underlying fragile health, citing traumatic brain injury from the automobile accident, being a victim of armed robberies with subsequent PTSD, and being suicidal. Ms. Harris also claimed intentional infliction of emotional distress, accusing Dr. Kreutzer of conducting behavior during the independent medical examination (IME) that was "intentionally designed to inflict emotional distress upon her or was done with reckless disregard for the consequences when he knew, or should have known, that emotional distress would result" [19]. She further claimed that his conduct was "outrageous" and her subsequent emotional distress was "severe."

The Supreme Court of Virginia found a "circumscribed duty" of forensic evaluators to their evaluees, a duty that is specifically limited to not harming the evaluee as a result of actual conduct of the examination. This duty, however limited, opens the door to malpractice claims. Forensic examiners should be aware that in certain jurisdictions, they are not strictly immune from malpractice claims stemming from court-ordered IMEs.

12.6   Conflicts of Interest

There are a number of potential conflicts of interest for the forensic mental health expert working in the judicial system. In various psychiatric malpractice cases, experts may be familiar with the defendant and should not accept the case where they have personal knowledge of the defendant. If asked by the defendant's attorney to help their friend, they should first speak with their colleague who is being sued to determine whether he or she indeed wants the mental health professional as their expert. Cross-examination could reveal bias toward the defendant by their expert because of prior knowledge and friendship. Certainly, if the mental health expert is asked by the plaintiff to attack their friend and colleague, they should refuse on the basis of prior relationship. Whenever an expert is asked to become involved in a case, he or she should immediately request the names of the principals in the case to determine whether or not there is a potential conflict of interest.

Another potential conflict of interest occurred in a civil case in which I had conducted an IME for the defense. I found the plaintiff was not malingering and that he had a legitimate illness following an injury. I discussed my opinion with the defense attorney, who understood my position and my opinions. I was surprised to then receive a telephone call from the plaintiff asking whether or not I could treat him after the legal case was over. I make it a point not to be available to treat those that I have evaluated, because I believe there is a potential conflict of interest. For example, if I was working for the plaintiff and helped the plaintiff receive an award of damages, I would not feel right about receiving part of that award for the treatment that I would then give to the patient. Similarly, I would not feel good about recommending an award for a patient that I was already treating, because that would be financially benefitting from my testimony. It is better in those cases to have an independent forensic psychiatrist to conduct the examination and make such a request that will not affect his or her income.

This case also underscores the fact that even though I was working for the defense, I was able, through judicious evaluation and testimony, to help the plaintiff receive the award he deserved. I was not an adversary who felt that he had to find no mental illness because I was working for the defense, which was their position.

12.7   Fees

Another area may involve the fees for work performed. Some experts believe that they are an essential part of the case and should be paid a percentage of the award. This, of course, has been found to be unethical as a contingency fee. Such fees may tend to color or distort the testimony in favor of the award. Some very well-known experts charge as much as US$1000 an hour for their work and feel they are worth it. Very few cases can pay such high fees, so the expert limits his or her work to those who can afford it. That being said, experts can charge whatever they wish knowing that they will be limiting their prospective clients. However, what is harmful to the professional and to forensic psychiatry is charging fees depending on what "the market will bear." Some experts will announce that they charge US$300 an hour for conducting an examination, reviewing records and preparing a report. However, they also announce that if they are called to court to testify or to deposition, they charge US$1000 for the first hour of the deposition, and US$750 per hour thereafter. Others will have a flat daily fee of either US$5000 or US$10 000 per day away from their practice. They justify such increase in hourly fees because they argue that the stress and strain of testimony and cross-examination warrants a higher remuneration. It is my opinion that it is more appropriate for the expert to have a single hourly rate for whatever he or she does in the field. One may increase one's hourly fee for testimony, but should disclose the difference to the attorney at the outset.

12.8   Harm under Cross-Examination

A number of psychiatrists do not like to have their opinions challenged in court, and many avoid forensic work like the plague, because they cannot tolerate the criticism that comes with the territory. Others wish to win cases, and when they do not, they feel as though they have failed, and they have let the retaining attorney down. That response depends upon the personality of the individual, and there are those in psychiatry perhaps, who should not be forensic experts, because they cannot tolerate losing, and also cannot tolerate having their opinions challenged.

A Caucasian psychiatrist had examined an African American woman who claimed she had been racially harassed and discriminated against at work. The plaintiff was complaining that she had serious emotional problems as a result of the harassment and discrimination. The psychiatrist was asked, on cross-examination by the plaintiff's attorney, whether she was a Negro, because she had evaluated a Negro woman who was racially harassed. The expert was flustered with that question, became defensive on the witness stand, saying that she is no more a Negro than was the expert who the plaintiff had called to examine his client. The question was meant by the plaintiff's attorney to throw the expert off balance and cause her to reconsider her position within the system. The question had its effect and the expert did not perform comfortably in court, becoming defensive and flustered.

I have always taught that the ideal expert is a teacher in court, and not an adversary. Experts can advocate for their side, but not become adversaries who argue when questioned. Experts should recognize that attorneys spend years learning how to ask proper questions and to chop holes in testimony by good cross-examination. Psychiatrists do not have this type of training. I have always advocated that it is not the expert's case to win or lose; it is the lawyer's responsibility. Ideally, the expert should have no interest in the outcome of the case.

I can attest that general psychiatric training does not prepare the average psychiatrist for forensic work. There are specialized training programs throughout the country that provide the kind of training one needs in order to survive and thrive in this field. That is why we recommend those who are interested in forensic work take a formal accredited training program with proper mentoring before entering the field where a brutal cross-examination may cause harm to our colleagues.

Gutheil [20] has written about his and others' experiences in court, and many of the irrelevant questions asked on cross-examination. A strong expert may disagree with the question asked and may refuse to answer the question on the ground that it is irrelevant. If the expert refuses, the court may order the expert to answer the question or be held in contempt. The expert feels there are some areas of privacy that he or she must maintain. For example, one expert was asked what his total income was for the previous year—that is, what he reported to the IRS. The expert said that was none of the attorney's business and he would not respond to that question. The court ordered him to respond, and he refused. The matter was taken on appeal, and the higher court upheld the expert's resisting to respond and explained to the sitting judge that the total income of the expert is not relevant to the case. What the expert made on that particular case, or even what the expert makes in doing forensic examinations and giving testimony may be relevant, but not his total income.

In their paper on "Narcissistic dimensions of expert witness practice," Gutheil and Simon [20] state, "The ideal embodiment of a witness free of narcissistic difficulties is the egoless expert who accepts that the task, not the person, is essential. This egoless state includes avoiding grandiosity, resisting the appeal of the limelight, avoiding taking personal credit for the outcome of the case, and avoiding gratuitously disparaging the opposing expert for one's own narcissistically competitive motives." The authors point out that the ego of some narcissistic experts can be harmful to the profession and to their case.

In another paper by Gutheil, Schetky, and Simon [21], "Fouling one's own nest," the authors give a number of case examples. One is about an expert who is asked about the reputation of an opposing expert who practiced in the same town. The authors state that experts should not respond to those questions because they are outside their mandate, or even their expertise. They suggest, "I have not been retained to assess another person's reputation but to give testimony on the matter at hand." Another response might be, "I have no factual data for such an opinion to a reasonable degree of medical certainty" [22].

In this paper, the authors present other conflicts of interest for the forensic psychiatrist. They are talking about institutional "nests" in which people belong to the same organization and criticize each other. The authors give the example of the psychiatrist who refused to become involved in a case involving a suicide in a prison where the plaintiff's attorney requested help. The expert turned down the request because he had previously worked as a staff psychiatrist at that prison and the defendant psychiatrist was a colleague of his. The same psychiatrist turned down another case where there was no such conflict except that he had worked at that prison, and he did not want to have a perception of bias [22].

The authors offer other examples of potential bias. They ask where one draws the line in accepting or refusing cases. They talk about special cases in which an expert witness observed the opposing expert, an individual from the same community that he regarded as a friend, sitting beside the cross-examining attorney and prompting the attorney in the cross-examination. (We have all done this, and I have recently refused to sit at counsel table because of the perception of bias.) The consulting expert, they state here, is in an ethical conflict with the testifying expert, who is supposed to be neutral and objective [22].

They note that sometimes attorneys will hire experts from the same department of psychiatry at a particular university in order to pit one professor from that university against another. It is wise to refuse such invitations.

The authors conclude that if one has to criticize a fellow local practitioner in a malpractice context, they recommend saying, "I am sorry to say that in this case Dr. X fell below the standard of care." They do not recommend trumpeting "This is the worst case of malpractice I have ever seen" [23]. Again, it is a matter of experts utilizing tact, sensitivity and common sense in court in order to avoid harm to themselves, to their colleagues, and to the profession. The authors summarize,

"Advocacy pressures and attorneys' needs and goals have the potential to bring out the worst in us, and we should resist ... Adhering to standards of appropriate conduct and mutual respect are the best safeguards against such fouling" [23].

12.9   Difficult Examinations

Sometimes, the forensic psychiatrist will be asked by a CEO of a major company to examine an employee, because the supervisors are concerned that he or she may "go postal." For example, an employee who has been making threats against other employees or, at a university, a professor who has written letters threatening colleagues who disagreed with his research. The employer indicates that the employee needs a psychiatric evaluation to determine whether he or she is "dangerous." It is my contention that unless one has great skill and experience in conducting these examinations, it is a dangerous thing to do for a novice forensic psychiatrist. The assessment of potential violent or self-destructive behavior is something that we do, but we should have some experience of doing it within the context of the employment or of the living situation. These individuals may prove to be "dangerous" to the examiners as well.

Another situation that may prove dangerous for the examiner is one in which a psychiatrist is asked whether or not a particular individual is competent to return to work. I am considering specifically a police officer who must carry a gun if he or she is competent to return to duty. In these cases, the assessing psychiatrist should demand immunity through one of the state or government agencies or be an employee of the government conducting such an examination. The situation may arise where psychiatrists conducting examinations are "damned if they do or damned if they don't." By that, I mean if he or she recommends the individual is competent to return to work and carry a weapon, and the officer misuses that weapon, the psychiatrist would be seen as wrong in making their prediction, and there will be some question whether the psychiatrist may be sued by the victim's family for recommending that the officer return to work and carry a gun when, clearly, he or she was not ready.

On the other hand, if the psychiatrist recommends the officer is still too unstable and would not recommend that he or she returns to duty carrying a gun, the officer may be relieved of duty and lose income. The officer may then sue to regain their position and may include the psychiatrist as a co-defendant in the lawsuit [24].

Unfortunately, there are some forensic psychiatrists who have their own problems with respect to various kinds of criminal behavior and are especially nasty to a defendant, for example, who is a child molester or who has killed or tortured children, and they can become downright insulting and hostile to the defendant, especially when working for the prosecution. Similarly, some psychiatrists cannot tolerate plaintiffs who malinger illness and they become nasty and hostile when examining such an individual for the defense. It is my opinion that these individuals who have such inherent biases create harmful situations for the examinee as well as for our profession and should not be involved in these cases. They damage the profession by their attitudes and their biases. Some of these psychiatrists commit intentional harm toward the examinee.

What of inadvertent or unintentional harm caused by unwitting or naïve examiners who should know better? They may not be aware that their probing questions will damage the individual or harm the examinee in some way.

A third category is what I have labeled "necessary collateral damage." That is, the questions that are asked of vulnerable individuals that need to be asked in order to determine facts or fantasies related to the legal issues at hand. Rape victims need to talk about the experience in order to determine their damages and their feelings. They need to talk about the nightmares, flashbacks, avoidance techniques, and hyper reactivity experiences in order for the examiner to document a proper diagnosis of PTSD.

In other situations, the defendant with multiple personality disorder or dissociative identity disorder needs to have the alters come forward in order to establish the diagnosis for legal purposes. Sometimes, the alter can create more damage when he or she emerges, and the examiner must be on guard. Sometimes, hypnosis or other forms of relaxation techniques will be utilized in order to bring forth the alternate personalities. Occasionally, that can be very destructive and harmful, but may be necessary.

Every forensic psychiatrist should understand the concept of risk factors in the work we do. Simon [25] has discussed risk factors in suicide and suggests we incorporate them as a standard of care. Malmquist's [26] book on homicide is similar, so that risk factors are enunciated, discussed, and put in place regarding the harm that may occur if the examination is incomplete, or without taking into account the various risk factors that are inherent in our work.

12.10   Judicial Bias Harming Defendant

In a case that was harmful because the judge appeared to have bias for the prosecution (since he had been the prosecutor in that jurisdiction prior to his ascending to the bench), I had examined an individual in a federal case for the defense, and could not help the defense. It became known that I did not write a report, and the prosecution subpoenaed me to testify in court not knowing what I was going to say, but believing it would be helpful to their side. I suggested that that would not be appropriate, because I had seen the man for the defense and worked under the attorney-client privilege for the defendant. The defense attorney appealed to the court to quash the subpoena, but the judge would not do so, and insisted that I testify, believing that I had seen the man for the defense and would give honest and valid testimony for the prosecution. I did testify under protest, since the judge ordered me to testify. After my testimony, the defendant was found guilty and was sentenced to a number of years in prison. On appeal, the Federal Court of Appeals criticized the judge, stating that he should never have forced me to testify since I had examined for the defense and it was not proper for the prosecution to call me as their expert, especially without the permission of the defense attorney. Thus, the defendant was harmed by my "forced testimony." It appears to me the difference is that a psychiatrist may testify for the defense even if he or she examined the defendant for the prosecution, because the prosecution is working for justice and truth, and the defense ethic is to defend the client as zealously as possible.

12.11   Boundary Crossing v. Boundary Violations

Gutheil [27] presents the distinction between boundary crossings and boundary violations. He notes boundary crossings may be unethical, but boundary violations may become criminal or approach legal difficulties. He states that boundary crossings are not always harmful to the patient in therapy, but boundary violations are. Boundary crossing may be hugging a needy patient, picking a patient up in a snowstorm and driving him or her, or offering help outside the traditional office situation. Gutheil indicates that the behavior should be discussed in the course of therapy so that there is a means for the patient to work through the change and the behavior between doctor and patient. However, the boundary violation involves extreme behavior or sexual behavior that the patient may volunteer or consent to, but because of the transference phenomenon, the behavior is harmful to the patient [27].

In forensic settings, the boundary issues are not as clear-cut as they are in treatment practice. The examiner indicates at the beginning of the session that this will not be a treatment session and there can be no treatment by the examiner. However, some examinations turn out to be therapeutic, and colleagues have indicated that there are times when they will offer advice to the examinee that they feel will be helpful for further improvement in their condition. They have given this advice irrespective of which side they are working for. Nevertheless, the examiner is not allowed to have boundary crossings or to have sex with the examinee or to assault the examinee [27]. The examiner is also not allowed to insult or criticize the examinee. Examiners are allowed to defend themselves or protect themselves from harm in the event that the examinee becomes violent.

12.12   Assessment of Dangerousness

When considering the issue of dangerousness, we do assess people to be "clear and present danger" of harm to themselves or others when considering involuntary commitment. We also evaluate when a person is no longer dangerous and thus is eligible to be discharged from a hospital. We also must assess whether our patient will act on his or her threat in Tarasoff [28] cases.

I have been concerned about psychiatrists rendering opinions about the dangerousness of mentally ill patients ever since the Tarasoff case in California in 1974 [29]. At that time the California Supreme Court gave the opinion that psychiatrists treating patients who commit violent acts toward third parties are liable for such acts if there was a communication in therapy that the patient was intending to harm an identifiable third party. This was known as the case of the "Duty to Warn," in which the psychiatrist had a duty to warn the intended victim of his patient's violence. That all presupposed, of course, that there was a doctor-patient relationship and that in the course of treatment, the patient told the psychiatrist of his intent and identified the third party who was to be harmed. The court opined that the "private privilege ends where the public peril begins" [29]. By that, it meant that because of the special relationship between the doctor and his patient, the doctor had a special duty to protect the third party who was under threat of harm by warning that person.

There were a number of protests to the Supreme Court ruling from the American Psychiatric Association and the California Psychiatric Society that led the California Supreme Court to rehear the case, and in 1976, the court came down with Tarasoff 2, which is a duty to protect rather than a duty to warn [28]. Since that time, there have been a number of progeny cases involving prediction of harm or violence, even toward property as well as toward persons [30].

Further, psychiatrists have been predicting dangerousness when the law changed with respect to committing patients to involuntary hospitalization. The former law that a person had to be mentally ill and in need of hospitalization was changed to mentally ill and a clear and present danger of harm to self or others. Thus, the psychiatrist committing a patient to the hospital or recommending to the court that the patient be committed, renders an opinion about the "dangerousness" of the patient.

Similarly, when patients who have been committed and treated and are ready to be released, the psychiatrist warrants to the community that the patient is no longer a danger to self or others. In a sense, he is predicting that the patient is currently "non-dangerous."

The notion of such changes occurred with the advent of mental health laws that gave mentally ill patients rights to lawyers, to court hearings, to due process of law when their freedom was curtailed. The idea, of course, is to protect the patient, but also to protect the community.

In juvenile decertification cases, the psychiatrist who recommends decertification from adult to juvenile court is warranting to the community that it is his or her opinion that this particular juvenile can be treated effectively in the juvenile system until the age of 21, so that when he or she comes out of confinement, they will not be a danger to the community.

Elsewhere, I have written about the pitfalls and perils in the practice of forensic psychiatry [24] and included the diagnosis of dangerousness as one of the potential areas of difficulty for forensic and other psychiatrists. I have given the recommendation that persons who are so committed should be committed because they are mentally ill and, under certain clinical conditions, are more likely to harm themselves or others, that is, to become violent or self-destructive. These are clinical terms that we can discuss rather than the legal concept of dangerousness, which has not been adequately defined and is clearly not a clinical term.

When discussing the issue of assessing a person for "dangerousness," Grisso and Tompkins [31] expressed guarded optimism regarding the progress being made in predicting future dangerousness:

> *When properly translated, the results of the new generation of violence risk studies might soon provide mental health professionals with a more reliable scientific foundation for describing the person's violence risk, thereby assisting society and deciding when these risks are sufficient to take action to protect a person and others. We have not yet achieved this capacity [31].*

Thus, it is my opinion that experts may do harm by giving opinions that are not based on scientific evidence. Zonana [32] criticizes the testimony given in sex offender cases, because of the need to testify that the person was "unable to control their behavior," which adds an additional dimension to the questions that experts may be asked. He cites the American Psychiatric Association's position statement on the insanity defense noting, "The difficulty in distinguishing an inability to control from a failure to control, analogizing it to distinguishing twilight from dusk" [32]. In summary, Zonana recommends that testimony about future dangerousness should not be given based on the Daubert/Kumho rulings [3,33]. He states, "Such testimony, lacking objective scientific testing or personal examination, defies scientific rigor and cannot be described as expert testimony. It is simply subject to testimony without any scientific validity by one who holds the medical degree" [34].

Zonana is concerned about the harm that can be caused when mental health experts give opinions in court without ever examining the defendant in a criminal case. He refers to the psychiatrist in Texas who testified in a number of capital sentencing cases, having arrived at his psychiatric diagnosis without examining the individuals in question and indicating while testifying as an expert witness that he could "predict with 100% certainty that the individuals would engage in future violent acts" [34].

In this instance, Zonana cites the case involving *Flores v. Johnson* [35] in which the expert witness psychiatrist did not examine Flores before testifying,

> *unequivocally that Flores would be a future danger, nor did he make his evaluation based on the psychological records or psychiatric testimony. Rather, he sat at trial and based his opinion on the facts of the offense and Flores' conduct during the trial (Flores did not testify). In this case not only did the expert testify that he could accurately predict the defendant's future dangerousness from a hypothetical, but he also told the jury that actually examining the defendant is 'a hindrance to a hypothetical question' [34].*

Another area in which psychiatrists predict the potential for future violence is in examining a defendant pre-trial to determine whether he or she is safe to be allowed out of confinement on bail. This may also be a very difficult problem for forensic psychiatrists inasmuch as their opinion, if followed, may lead to harm to the defendant if they are released and become violent, or if they are not released and must remain in confinement until their trial.

There are a variety of contexts in which predictions are made about a patient's acting in ways that endanger others. Civil commitment statutes allow for involuntary commitment when a patient, as a result of his or her mental illness, is a clear and present danger to self or others. Also, sentencing statutes allow psychiatrists to examine patients to see whether they have a propensity for violent behavior. Offenders with diagnosed personality disorders may receive greater punishments, especially if they are labeled as having an antisocial personality disorder or as a psychopath.

Psychiatrists are also called upon by the courts to determine the potential for a patient to commit further "dangerous" acts. The Tarasoff case has placed a duty upon psychiatrists to protect potential victims from their patients' violent acts. Also, psychiatrists who discharge patients from hospitals where the patient later commits a violent act, face the threat of liability for releasing the patient "prematurely" from the hospital.

As early as 1974, a Task Force of the American Psychiatric Association concluded that "The state of the art regarding predictions of violence is very unsatisfactory. The ability of psychiatrists or any other professionals to reliably predict future violence is unproved" [36].

An unofficial statement by the American Psychiatric Association in 1983 on the prediction of dangerousness, reported that

> *We have previously noted the limitations of predicting violence. Considerable evidence has been accumulated by now to demonstrate the long term predictions by psychiatrists of future violence is an extremely inaccurate process. The most that can be said about any individual is that a history of past violence increases the probability that future violence will occur ... In addition the psychiatrist may well wish to comment on factors in the individual's environment that are likely to increase (e.g., alcohol, rejection by a girlfriend) or decrease (e.g., taking psychotropic medication) the probability of future violence [37].*

Legal statutes have mandated that we predict future dangerousness, especially in commitment procedures and when releasing patients from hospitals. We psychiatrists do have limitations on our ability to make such predictions; however, studies have shown that certain diagnostic categories have a greater propensity for violence. The MacArthur studies show that if one mixes alcohol or substance abuse with a psychotic diagnosis, the likelihood of future violent behavior increases [38].

Nevertheless, I would recommend we remove the word "dangerousness" from our predictions since we are not experts on the prediction of dangerousness, or even in the diagnosis of it. (Of course, there is no diagnosis of dangerousness.) Even the definition of dangerousness is difficult and fraught with problems for the forensic psychiatrist. Rather, I would recommend that we substitute the word "violent behavior," which is observable or "self-destructive behavior," which is also observable. They are both clinical behaviors that we can observe and discuss prediction of such behavior under certain clinical conditions, including past similar behavior. In the context of this book, it is my opinion that making such predictions without clear clinical evidence can be harmful to the individual about whom we predict and may even be harmful to others in the community, to our profession and to ourselves.

12.13   Summary

In summary, there are a number of risks forensic experts take when undertaking their responsibility in assessing, report writing, and testifying. They may be liable for inappropriate behavior during the conduct of an examination or by putting inappropriate comments in a report. They may also be subject to inappropriate cross-examination during testimony that could be harmful to them. The vagaries of the judicial system may also impinge upon forensic experts causing harm to them and to their subjects.

Predicting dangerousness can be a particular "danger" for the forensic psychiatrist. This chapter is meant to alert the forensic expert to those dangers of practicing forensic psychiatry that may negatively affect him or her. Thus, the forensic expert becomes a vulnerable individual as well as others noted in other chapters of this book. By adhering to the ethical guidelines of AAPL and adhering to "Minimizing harm to the subject," we will be in a better position to reduce the risk of harm to ourselves.

References

1. Weinstock, R. and Garrick, T. (1995) Is liability possible for forensic psychiatrists? *Bulletin of the American Academy of Psychiatry and the Law*, **23**, 183–93.
2. Binder, R. (2002) Liability for the psychiatrist expert witness. *The American Journal of Psychiatry*, **159**(11), 1819–25.
3. *Daubert v. Merrill Dow Pharmaceuticals*, 509 US 579, 113 Sup. Ct. 2786, (1993).
4. *Briscoe v. LaHue*, 460 US 325, (1983).
5. *Mitchell v. Forsyth*, 472 US 511, (1985).
6. *Levine v. Wiss & Co.*, 478 A.2d 397, (1984).
7. *Pettus v. Cole et al.*, 49 Cal. App. 4th 402, (1996).
8. *Murphy v. A.A. Matthews*, 841 SW.2d 671, (1992).
9. See Ref. [2], p. 1824.
10. Federation of State Medical Boards, at: www.fsmb.org
11. American Medical Association, at: www.AMA.org
12. American Psychiatric Association (2008) *The Principles of Medical Ethics With Annotations Especially Applicable to Psychiatry*, Washington DC.
13. Leavitt, N., Presskreischer, H., Maykuth, P.L. and Grisso, T. (2006) Aggression toward forensic evaluators: A statewide survey. *Journal of the American Academy of Psychiatry and the Law*, **34**, 231–9.
14. Miller, R.D. (1985) The harassment of forensic psychiatrists outside of court. *Bulletin of the American Academy of Psychiatry and the Law*, **13**, 337–43.
15. See Ref. [14], p. 342.

16. Kroll, J. and Mackenzie, T.B. (1983) When psychiatrists are liable: risk management and violent patients. *Hospital and Community Psychiatry*, **34**, 29–35.

17. Petrilla, J. and Sadoff, R.L. (1992) Confidentiality and the family as caregiver. *Hospital and Community Psychiatry*, **43**(2), 136–9.

18. Gutheil, T.G. (1998) *The Psychiatrist in Court: A Survival Guide*, American Psychiatric Press, Washington DC.

19. *Harris v. Kreutzer*, 624 SE.2d 24 (Va. 2006).

20. Gutheil, T.G. and Simon, R.I. (2005) Narcissistic dimensions of expert witness practice. *Journal of the American Academy of Psychiatry and the Law*, **33**, 55–8.

21. Gutheil, T.G., Schetky, D.H., and Simon, R.I. (2006) Pejorative testimony about opposing experts and colleagues: "Fouling one's own nest". *Journal of the American Academy of Psychiatry and the Law*, **34**, 26–30.

22. See Ref. [21], p. 29.

23. See Ref. [21], p. 30.

24. Sadoff, R.L. (1998) The practice of forensic psychiatry: perils, problems and pitfalls. *Journal of the American Academy of Psychiatry and the Law*, **26**, 305–14.

25. Simon, R.I. (2004) *Assessing and Managing Suicide Risk: Guidelines for Clinically Based Risk Management*, American Psychiatric Press, Washington, DC.

26. Malmquist, C.P. (2006) *Homicide: A Psychiatric Perspective*, 2nd edn, American Psychiatric Press, Washington, DC.

27. Gutheil, T.G. (2008) Boundary Crossings v. Boundary Violations. *Psychiatric Times*, p. 28.

28. *Tarasoff v. Regents of the University of California*, 17 Cal.3d 425; 551 P.2d 334; 131 Cal. Rptr. 14, (1976).

29. *Tarasoff v. Regents of the University of California et al.*, 529 P.2d 553, (1974).

30. (a)*Thompson v. County of Alameda*, 27 Cal.3d 741; 614 P.2d 728; 167 Cal. Rptr. 70, (1980); (b) *Brady v. Hopper*, 570 F. Supp. 1333, (D. Colo. 1983); (c) *Peterson v. State*, 100 Wash. 2d 421; 671 P.2d 230, (1983); (d) *Jablonski by Pahls v. United States*, 712 F.2d 391 (9th Cir. 1983); (e) *Hamman v. County of Maricopa*, 775 P.2d 1122 (Ariz. 1989).

31. Grisso, T. and Tompkins, A.J. (1996) Communicating violence risk assessments. *American Journal of Psychology*, **51**, 928–30.

32. Zonana, H. (2000) Sex offender testimony: junk science or unethical testimony? *The Journal of the American Academy of Psychiatry and the Law*, **28**, 386–8.

33. *Kumho Tire Co. v. Carmichael*, 526 US 137, (1999).

34. See Ref. [32], p. 388.

35. *Flores v. Johnson*, 210 F.3d 456, (5th Cir. 2000).

36. American Psychiatric Association (1974) Task Force Report No. 8, Washington, DC.

37. American Psychiatric Association (1983) Statement on the Prediction of Dangerousness, press release dated March 18, 1983.

38. The MacArthur Violence Risk Assessment Study. See links: http://www.Macarthur.Virginia.edu/violence.html and http://www.Macarthur.Virginia.edu/risk.html (accessed June 11, 2010).

13 Risks of Harm to the Forensic Expert: the Legal Perspective

Donna L. Vanderpool

Professional Risk Management Services, Inc., Arlington, VA, USA

13.1 Introduction

Forensic activities have the potential to harm the individual who is the subject of the forensic activity, and the harm alleged by a subject has the potential to harm the forensic psychiatrist. The consequences of this alleged harm are increasing, as there is more interest in evaluating and holding physicians accountable for forensic activities. For example, courts have begun to depart from the traditional rule of not imposing liability on physicians in forensic activities, and state medical boards and professional associations have become more active in reviewing these activities. This chapter focuses on the liability of psychiatrists for harm alleged in forensic work—specifically, performing independent medical evaluations (IMEs) and providing expert witness testimony.

Note that although many cases are discussed in this chapter, case law related to liability for forensic activities is still developing, and, in fact, relevant case law is non-existent in many jurisdictions. Uniformity is lacking among the cases that do exist; accordingly, the fact that a case is discussed here does not mean that another similar case with a different outcome does not exist or will not exist in the future. What follows is a brief overview of the issues in this evolving area of liability.

13.2 Harm From IME Activities

Dissatisfied evaluees have several avenues of complaint available to them, such as filing a lawsuit and/or triggering regulatory agency investigations (e.g., state

Disclaimer: Nothing in this chapter is to be construed as or relied upon as legal advice.

Ethical Issues in Forensic Psychiatry: Minimizing Harm   by Robert L. Sadoff
© 2011 John Wiley & Sons, Ltd

medical boards for all types of complaints and the Department of Health and Human Services for violations of the Privacy and Security Rules under the Health Insurance Portability and Accountability Act (HIPAA). When suing a forensic physician, evaluees have many civil causes of action to choose from, and they often allege medical malpractice.

A plaintiff must prove all four of the following elements to win a medical malpractice lawsuit: (i) duty (defendant physician owed plaintiff the duty to meet the standard of care), (ii) negligence (defendant failed to meet that duty/standard of care), (iii) damages, and (iv) causation (plaintiff's damages were caused by defendant's negligence). Application of these elements, however, is not always straightforward in IME cases.

13.2.1   Duty Owed to the Evaluee and Liability for Medical Malpractice

Courts seem to agree that the physician's duty in performing an IME is not the same as the duty owed to the physician's patients. The courts disagree, however, on what exact duty, if any, the physician does owe the evaluee. Traditionally courts have held that physicians engaged in forensic activities cannot be held liable for malpractice because there is no physician-patient relationship. Without a treatment relationship, there can be no duty owed to the evaluee; without a duty there can be no breach; and without a breach, there can be no liability. However, psychiatrists should not assume that just because there is no patient-psychiatrist relationship, that there is no duty owed to the evaluee. Courts are reexamining this issue, with some courts recognizing a "limited" patient-physician relationship for IME purposes. The Kansas Supreme Court in *Smith v. Welch* [1] summarized the issue of the physician's duty of care while performing IMEs by noting the following from the Colorado Supreme Court:

> *Many courts set forth a 'general' rule that in the absence of a physician-patient relationship a physician owes no duty to an examinee. Many of these same courts, however, recognize a duty of care if the examining physician undertakes in some way to act on behalf of the examinee or induces reasonable reliance by the person examined. Some courts conclude that medical malpractice standards govern, and recognize a duty of care simply on the basis of the relationship created by the referral and examination. Others agree but temper this conclusion by expressly limiting the scope of the duty to the functions the physician agrees to undertake. Still others hold that the absence of a physician-patient relationship precludes a malpractice action, with the concomitant broad duty of care, but that an ordinary negligence action can be maintained in appropriate circumstances. Some of these latter cases are based on the well recognized principle that a person who assumes to act must act with care.*

For a more in-depth analysis of the various state views on the requirement of a physician-patient relationship for liability, see *Stanley v. McCarver* [2]. In this case, the majority opinion by the Arizona Supreme Court acknowledged that the requirement of a physician-patient relationship has been "quietly eroding in several jurisdictions," and held that "the absence of a formal doctor-patient relationship does not necessarily preclude the imposition of a duty of care." There was also a dissenting opinion discussing the contrary case law.

Case law indicates that the following duties may be expected: the duty not to injure the evaluee, the duty to properly diagnose, the duty to inform, and the duty to protect confidentiality.

13.2.1.1   First Possible Duty—the Duty Not to Injure the Evaluee During the Examination

Most courts agree that, even if there is no other duty, the examining physician has the duty to avoid physically injuring the evaluee during the examination. This has been true even in courts following the traditional rule that IMEs do not create a physician-patient relationship. This duty not to injure the evaluee can encompass both mental and physical harm. As noted in a footnote by the Colorado Supreme Court in *Martinez v. Lewis* [3]:

> It is entirely possible that a duty of care could arise while a physician or other health care provider conducts an evaluation of an examinee's mental health. For instance, if the physician or other health care provider conducted an evaluation in a manner that worsened the examinee's mental health and the physician or other health care provider knew or should have known about information that would have cautioned against conducting the examination in that manner, a duty might well arise.

The issue of mental harm to the forensic evaluee came before the Virginia Supreme Court in *Harris v. Kreutzer* [4]. The court ruled that a doctor who conducts an IME of a party in litigation has no duty to diagnose or treat the examinee, and no liability may arise from the doctor's report or testimony regarding the exam, because the doctor's duty is solely to examine the party without harming her in conducting the evaluation. However, the court went on to say that a malpractice action *may* lie for negligent performance of the examination. In this case, the evaluee alleged that during the IME, the psychologist had "verbally abused [her], raised his voice to her, caused her to break down into tears in his office, stated she was putting on a show, and accused her of being a faker and malingerer." Plaintiff also alleged "that despite his knowledge of her condition, [he] intentionally aggravated her pre-existing condition and her post-traumatic stress disorder and her brain injury." Accordingly, she alleged that the psychologist breached his duty to her in conducting the IME because he "failed to appropriately examine and evaluate [her] mental status ... and was deliberately abusive with disregard for the consequences of his conduct," and as a result, the plaintiff alleged that her mental and physical health "drastically deteriorated." The court dismissed the claim of intentional infliction of emotional distress and remanded the case back to the trial court to determine if the psychologist breached his duty not to harm the evaluee in the performance of the IME.

It is important to note that courts have not generally found an adverse outcome or loss stemming from an IME physician's report to be an adequate basis for a lawsuit. As stated by the Michigan Supreme Court in *Dyer v. Trachtman* [5], "the

IME physician, acting at the behest of a third party, is not liable to the examinee for damages resulting from the conclusions the physician reaches or reports."

13.2.1.2   Second Possible Duty—the Duty to Properly Diagnose

Courts that impose this duty are currently in the minority. However, in at least one case—*Lambely v. Kameny* [6]—an appellate court found that a psychiatrist who performed an IME for an employer had a duty to diagnose with reasonable professional skill, even though the traditional doctor-patient relationship did not exist.

13.2.1.3   Third Possible Duty—the Duty to Inform the Evaluee About a Potentially Serious Medical Condition

In addition to being imposed by the majority of courts, this duty is found in the AMA Ethics Opinion E-10.03 *Patient-Physician Relationship in the Context of Work-Related and Independent Medical Examinations* (1999). Also, state medical boards may impose the obligation to disclose. For example, the New Jersey Medical Board regulation 13:35-6.5 requires "that should the examination disclose abnormalities or conditions not known to the examinee, the licensee shall advise the examinee to consult another health care professional for treatment."

Psychiatrists are encouraged to disclose by informing the evaluee directly. In at least one case—*Reed v. Bojarski* [7]—this duty to inform was found to be non-delegable, even where the contract with the third party stated that the third party would notify the examinee. Accordingly, psychiatrists should ensure that all contracts for IMEs allow the evaluating physician to inform the evaluee directly of any serious medical conditions.

13.2.1.4   Fourth Possible Duty—the Duty to Maintain Confidentiality

This duty of confidentiality owed—even when no treatment is provided—is recognized in case law and is the majority view. This duty is also required by state and federal laws, including 42 CFR Part 2 related to confidentiality of drug and alcohol treatment records and HIPAA regulations. The duty of confidentiality is also imposed by various ethics codes, including the AMA's Ethics Opinion 5.09 *Confidentiality: Industry-Employed Physicians and Independent Medical Examiners* (1999).

State confidentiality law is also relevant to forensic psychiatrists. In *Pettus v. Cole* [8], the appellate court held that two IME psychiatrists violated state confidentiality law when they disclosed to the employer information from the evaluation they performed at the employer's request. Although state law required an authorization to release, both IME psychiatrists discussed with the employer—without authorization—the evaluee's alcohol use. Based on the IME reports, the employer required the evaluee to complete an inpatient alcohol treatment program as a condition of his return to work. The employee refused and was fired. He then sued both IME psychiatrists and the employer. The trial court granted the psychiatrists' motion for judgment on both allegations (violation of confidentiality statute and invasion of his constitutional right of privacy). Plaintiff appealed, and the appellate court found that both psychiatrists had violated the confidentiality statute.

For psychiatrists who are covered providers under HIPAA, the Privacy Rule's requirements apply to all disclosures of protected health information, regardless of the purpose for which the protected health information was created. Once a provider meets the regulatory definition of a health care provider subject to the HIPAA regulations, then that provider must comply with the Privacy Rule's requirements for *all* uses and disclosures of protected health information.

To assist covered providers in fulfilling this legal obligation, the Privacy Rule has an exception for IME physicians to the general rule that treatment cannot be conditioned upon the individual signing an authorization for the disclosure of information [9].

Accordingly, IME physicians are expressly allowed to require the evaluee to sign an authorization for the release of protected health information to the third party requesting the IME as a condition of performing the IME.

In addition, the Office for Civil Rights (which enforces the Privacy Rule) has made it clear in its published enforcement cases that a medical practice was wrong to deny the individual a copy of the medical records after performing an IME on behalf of an insurance company [10].

13.2.2   What About Immunity?

There can be immunity from suit for some forensic activities, and it is this immunity that has led to greater scrutiny of forensic activities by licensing boards and professional organizations. There are two types of immunity relevant to forensic psychiatrists:

1. **Quasi-judicial immunity** (for persons other than judges when performing judicial activities) protects the evaluator's *performance of judicial activities*. As noted by the appellate court in *Awai v. Kotin* [11], performing evaluations and making recommendations are activities "intimately related and essential to the judicial process of finding facts and rendering decisions" so that quasi-judicial immunity may be available for these activities. However, note that this immunity is generally only available when the IME provider is retained by and reports directly to the court.
2. **Witness immunity** provides immunity from suit only for testimony in a judicial proceeding, which can include a deposition. This immunity generally precludes claims based on statements, opinions, or findings set forth in a report or testimony, but it will not preclude a complaint based on the physician's actions in conducting a forensic evaluation and preparing a report.

The case law discussing immunity for IMEs shows that immunity available to IME physicians varies with the type of IME.

13.2.2.1   IME Physician Retained for Purposes Other Than Litigation

Without activities in the judicial context, there can be no judicial immunity or witness immunity.

13.2.2.2   IME Physician Retained by a Party for Litigation Purposes

Most courts find that there is no quasi-judicial immunity for an IME physician's activities where he or she performs an examination at the request of a party, even if the court enters an order authorizing the IME. Quasi-judicial immunity is generally available only where the examiner is retained by, and reports directly to the court. However, witness immunity may be available. As long as the examination is performed for litigation, and in anticipation of the examiner testifying regarding the examination, the physician generally has absolute witness immunity. Accordingly, claims based on any statements, opinions, or findings that are set forth in any report or in any testimony (whether in deposition or in trial) are generally precluded.

13.2.2.3   IME Physician Retained by the Court for Evaluation and Recommendations

In addition to possible witness immunity, where the court retains an expert for the evaluation of claims or otherwise, quasi-judicial immunity generally protects the expert for activities related to the judicial process of finding facts and rendering decisions. As noted by the Utah Supreme Court in *Parker v. Dodgion* [12], "courts ... have uniformly held that psychologists appointed by the court to conduct psychological evaluations of parties involved in custody disputes perform a function integral to the judicial process and are therefore immune from suit" and such quasi-judicial immunity means that "even if [the evaluator] was in fact negligent in the way he conducted his court-appointed duties, he is nonetheless entitled to immunity." Note, however, that this immunity is contingent on the IME physician actually being appointed by the court. In *Politi v. Tyler* [13], the Supreme Court of Vermont found that the trial court's order stating "[f]orensic evaluation will be done" and "counsel to let us know within a week who to engage for a forensic evaluation" was held not to be sufficient to categorize defendant psychiatrist in subsequent malpractice case as a court appointed expert entitled to immunity.

In *Dalton v. Miller* [14], the Colorado Court of Appeals addressed many of these points about immunity. Plaintiff Dalton sued her insurance company, and the insurance company hired a psychiatrist to perform an IME. The psychiatrist examined the plaintiff, prepared a written report for the insurance company, and gave a deposition. The plaintiff settled her case against the insurance company and then sued the psychiatrist alleging (i) that the psychiatrist's conduct during the IME harmed her and (ii) that there had been misrepresentation related to alleged discrepancies between the psychiatrist's written report and his testimony. The court dismissed both claims based on the psychiatrist's immunity. The appellate court reversed in part. The court upheld the dismissal related to discrepancies between the report and testimony holding that the physician had witness immunity for testimony, including depositions and reports. The appellate court remanded part of the case back to the trial court because the IME physician may have had a duty to avoid causing the evaluee harm during the actual examination. There was no judicial immunity because the IME provider was not appointed by the court.

13.2.3   Licensing Board Actions

Anyone, including IME evaluees, can file a complaint with the evaluator's licensing board. Filing a board complaint can be an appealing option to evaluees and other third parties for several reasons. Specifically, there is no requirement of damages (as is the case with lawsuits), there is no statute of limitations within which the complaint has to be filed, and medical boards generally investigate all complaints received no matter how meritless they appear to be. The risk of an unhappy evaluee filing a board complaint is considerable, and this risk is even greater when performing custody evaluations, where at least one parent is likely to be unhappy with the evaluation.

13.2.4   Liability Points—Performing IMEs

1. Harm claimed by an evaluee allegedly caused by the forensic psychiatrist can include mental harm.
2. The trend by courts is to impose liability without the traditional physician-patient relationship.
3. Generally, these duties, at least, will be found to be owed to the evaluee: to not injure the evaluee, to disclose information about a serious medical condition to the evaluee, and to maintain confidentiality.
4. Judicial immunity will likely apply only if the psychiatrist is actually retained by the court (not just retained by a party per court order).
5. Providers covered under HIPAA's Privacy Rule have exposure for breach of confidentiality, even with IME evaluees.
6. Anyone can file a licensing board complaint.

13.2.5   Risk Management Advice—Performing IMEs

1. Understand the duties owed to the evaluee.
2. Manage the evaluee's expectations so that it is clear that the IME is being done at the request of a third party and that there is no treatment relationship.
3. Documentation is especially useful—it may be prudent to have evaluees sign a consent form spelling things out.
4. Inform the evaluee of significant medical findings.

13.3   Harm From Expert Witness Testimony

Liability exposure for expert witness activities can be divided into four categories: (i) civil litigation, (ii) criminal prosecution, (iii) discipline by licensing boards, and (iv) peer review and discipline by professional organizations. Additionally, disciplinary actions, malpractice settlements and judgments, and sanctions by professional associations are reportable to the National Practitioner Data Bank.

13.3.1 Civil Litigation Against Experts

As discussed above, most states recognize witness immunity to preclude liability from statements made in judicial proceedings. Reasons for allowing witness immunity include the following: the expert's testimony is under oath, the expert is subject to cross-examination, and there is the threat of criminal prosecution for perjury. However, witness immunity only provides immunity from a lawsuit—not immunity from investigation by a licensing board or professional association.

13.3.1.1 Litigation Against Adverse Expert

In terms of litigation brought by a party adverse to the expert, courts generally have found that witness immunity precludes claims against adverse experts. As stated in an opinion from the California Attorney General [15], "when a physician testifies as an expert in a civil proceeding regarding the standard of medical care ... the physician may not, on the basis of his or her testimony, be held liable in a subsequent tort action brought by the adverse party." The opinion also states that the expert may be subject to discipline by the state medical board.

Having said that courts generally find witness immunity precludes suit against adverse experts, there still continue to be cases filed against adverse experts. Given witness immunity, these plaintiffs typically plead very creative causes of action. In *MacGregor v. Rutberg* [16], a neurosurgeon sued the expert who testified for the patient in a medical malpractice lawsuit, alleging defamation, and breach of contract. The trial court dismissed the case and the dismissal was affirmed on appeal. The appellate court held that on the defamation claim, the expert had absolute immunity from defamation based on his testimony. The court also dismissed the breach of contract claim. Plaintiff (defendant neurosurgeon in the underlying medical malpractice claim) alleged that at the time of the expert testimony, the expert witness was a member of the American Association of Neurological Surgeons (AANS), which had rules related to members' expert testimony. Plaintiff claimed that by joining AANS, the expert waived absolute witness immunity by agreeing to abide by rules that regulate members' testimony. The court noted that although the organization itself can enforce its own rules, members are not allowed to enforce the rules against each other.

In *Wilson v. Bernet* [17], the plaintiff, who was very unhappy with the expert psychiatrist's testimony in a custody case, did not even bother pleading in terms of the testimony. Instead, the plaintiff asserted a cause of action for tortious interference with a parental relationship. The Supreme Court of West Virginia held that "no cause of action for tortious interference with parental or custodial relationship may be maintained against an adverse expert witness based upon his/her expert testimony and/or participation in a custody proceeding."

13.3.1.2   Litigation Against Friendly Expert

There have been cases where a party sued its own expert. Most of these cases involved financial errors by the expert [18,19]. In *Marrogi v. Howard* [20], the Louisiana Supreme Court held that witness immunity does not bar a claim "against a retained expert witness, asserted by a party who in prior litigation retained that expert, which claim arises from the expert's allegedly deficient performance of his duties to provide litigation services, such as the formulation of opinions and recommendations, and to give opinion testimony before or during trial."

Pace v. Swerdlow [21] involved an expert who changed his mind right before trial and was sued. The facts are as follows: the plaintiffs hired a physician to serve as their expert witness in a medical malpractice case related to their daughter's death following plastic surgery. Very close to trial, the expert was deposed. In his deposition, when asked about testifying without having seen the defendant's deposition transcript, the expert replied "I think it would have been good for me to have seen it, and I did not ask for it. I did not think to ask for it." The expert also admitted that he had never testified in trial, and that he was "a relative novice at this whole thing." Following his deposition, he reviewed the anesthesiologist's depositions. When he received a copy of his own deposition transcript, he (without consulting the attorney that retained him) drafted a two-page "Addendum" that directly opposed plaintiff's malpractice claims and supported the anesthesiologist's defense. Defendant physicians then moved for summary judgment. The court granted summary judgment for the defendant physicians. Instead of appealing this decision, the plaintiffs filed suit against the expert in federal court alleging professional malpractice, fraud, negligent misrepresentation, breach of fiduciary duty, breach of contract, breach of implied covenant of good faith and fair dealing, and negligent infliction of emotional distress. The expert filed a motion to dismiss claiming witness immunity. The federal trial court granted the expert's motion to dismiss all claims holding that plaintiffs' loss was not caused by any alleged change in opinion by the expert. Plaintiffs appealed, and the federal appellate court agreed with plaintiff and held that the expert *may* have proximately caused the plaintiffs to have their case dismissed prematurely. The appellate court reversed and remanded the case back to trial court, noting that the expert could address the issue of immunity with the trial court.

13.3.1.3   Litigation Against a Court-Appointed Expert

In *Levine v. Wiss & Co.* [22], the New Jersey Supreme Court allowed litigation against a purportedly court-appointed accountant who was allegedly negligent in valuing business assets. Although it is not clear from the opinion if the expert was actually appointed by the court, the court stated that "a court appointment is not a talisman for immunity. It does not alter the critical fact that defendants exercised no quasi-judicial power" and therefore are not entitled to immunity from charges of negligence.

13.3.1.4 Litigation Against a Medical Board's Expert

Kobrin v. Gastfriend [23] involved suit against an expert retained by the licensing board to investigate a complaint. The expert stated that the standard of care had not been met. The board brought disciplinary action against the physician but later exonerated the physician of all charges. The physician then sued the board's expert for expert witness malpractice, defamation, malicious prosecution, and intentional interference with contractual relations. The expert moved to dismiss, asserting immunity under the state anti-SLAPP (Strategic Lawsuit Against Public Participation) statute, which is tied to a citizen's right to petition the government. The trial court agreed with the expert and granted the expert's motion to dismiss. The plaintiff appealed to the state Appeals Court, but the Massachusetts Supreme Court instead decided to hear the case. The state Supreme Court disagreed with the expert and held the statue did not apply, as there was no petitioning here—the defendant "was acting solely on behalf of the medical board as an expert." The case was remanded back down to the trial court to address regular witness immunity.

Fortunately, as indicated by the federal trial court in *Kutilek v. Gannon* [24], "consultants and advisors to administrative boards have been protected from damage suits on the basis of absolute immunity."

13.3.2 Criminal Prosecution

Criminal charges against experts are extremely rare in medical malpractice cases; perjury is difficult to prove, especially when it is related to a medical opinion. However, criminal charges can be brought and can involve more than perjury—charges can also include mail fraud and wire fraud. For example, a Florida surgeon was indicted for false testimony [25]. The surgeon had testified for a patient who sued a Veterans Administration hospital. The US Attorney's office defended the hospital in the case. The criminal indictment charged that the physician falsely testified that he was the lead surgeon in an average of 10–12 coronary bypass graft procedures per year in the six years leading up to the case when, in fact, he had performed none for the several years prior to his testimony. In addition to the perjury allegation, the indictment also alleged that he used the US mail and interstate communications to defraud a plaintiff who relied on his testimony in a malpractice case in Oakland, and alleged that he gave false testimony during a deposition in another malpractice case in Detroit.

A plea agreement was reached [26], and the surgeon pled guilty to contempt of court, which carries a maximum sentence of one year. In addition to paying restitution, the surgeon also agreed to retire and to publish a letter in a professional medical journal acknowledging his offense and his responsibility for it, and the consequences of that offense to him and to the administration of justice.

13.3.3 Licensing Board Issues

13.3.3.1 Licensing Board Actions

Providing expert witness testimony can constitute the practice of medicine, even if there is no physician-patient relationship and no treatment is provided, at least according to the AMA, the Federation of State Medical Boards, individual state medical boards, and at least one appellate case, *Joseph v. District of Columbia Board of Medicine* [27]. The significance of having the practice of medicine defined to include providing expert testimony is that the expert's activities are subject to regulation and oversight by the state. Consequences of this regulation by the state licensing body could include disciplinary action, litigation to fight the disciplinary action, National Practitioner Data Bank reporting, and loss of business.

Even if providing expert testimony is not considered the practice of medicine, states may still have the ability to regulate experts and discipline a physician for professional misconduct. After stating that this is true in California, the California Attorney General (in the previously referenced opinion [15]) went on to state that "conceivably, such misconduct would include court testimony given on behalf of a plaintiff or defendant as to the appropriate standard of medical care and whether the defendant has breached that standard."

One of the most well-known cases involving a medical board's discipline related to expert testimony is *In re Lustgarten* [28]. Dr. Lustgarten's license was revoked by the North Carolina Medical Board based on a finding that he engaged in unprofessional conduct by misstating in testimony facts and the appropriate standard of care. Dr. Lustgarten appealed this decision and the trial court reversed five of the board's six grounds for discipline. The court affirmed one of the board's findings, holding that the doctor's testimony that a doctor in the case had falsified records was not a protected opinion. The court sent the case back to the board for a disciplinary hearing on that one issue. The board then changed the doctor's punishment from revocation of his license to a one-year revocation, which the doctor continued to fight. This one-year revocation was upheld by the court. Dr. Lustgarten appealed again and the North Carolina Court of Appeals finally agreed with Dr. Lustgarten and found "substantial evidence of record demonstrates that he had a good faith basis" for his testimony and ordered the disciplinary charges be dismissed.

13.3.3.2 Regulation of Expert Testimony

States have enacted various statutes and regulations addressing expert testimony. For example, the Kansas legislature enacted statute 60-3412, which states that "in any medical malpractice liability action ... no person shall qualify as an expert witness ... unless at least 50% of such person's professional time within the two-year period preceding the incident giving rise to the action is devoted to actual clinical practice in the same profession in which the defendant is licensed." Another example is the Mississippi Medical Board; Chapter 22 of the Medical Board's Rules and Regulations has various provisions making physicians who testify as experts more accountable for their testimony. There are also specific requirements in these regulations for out-of-state experts. If these requirements are not followed, the out-of-state expert could be accused of practicing without a license, which could result in civil and criminal penalties, as well as possibly voiding the malpractice insurance coverage.

13.3.4   Discipline by Professional Organizations

In addition to regulation by medical boards, forensic psychiatrists are subject to peer review and discipline by professional organizations such as the APA [29], AMA [30], and state medical associations. One well-known case involving regulation of experts by professional associations is *Austin v. AANS* [31]. Dr. Austin sued his specialty society, claiming it unfairly suspended him in retaliation for testifying for a plaintiff—and against fellow AANS member—in a malpractice case. AANS said the suspension was based on "unprofessional testimony." The trial court stated that it did not have the power to interfere with the internal operations of a private association. Dr. Austin appealed the decision and the Seventh Circuit Court of Appeals held that a professional society was allowed to suspend a member after a hearing showed that he had given improper testimony as an expert witness at a medical malpractice trial. The court further found that Dr. Austin had violated the Association's Code of Ethics and witness guidelines, he was provided due process by AANS, and he had failed to show that AANS had substantially impaired his economic interest. Dr. Austin appealed again. The US Supreme Court denied Dr. Austin's request to hear the case, so the ruling from the Court of Appeals that a professional society can discipline a member concerning expert testimony stood.

Another case involving a professional organization investigating a physician's testimony is *Fullerton v. Florida Medical Ass'n. Inc.* [32] Dr. Fullerton was an expert witness for the plaintiff in a medical malpractice case, which plaintiff ultimately lost. The defendants (who won) then asked the Florida Medical Association (FMA) to review Dr. Fullerton's expert testimony. Dr. Fullerton then sued the three complaining physicians and the FMA alleging defamation, tortious interference with advantageous business relationships, conspiracy, and witness intimidation. The trial court ruled that the FMA and the individual physicians had immunity under a Florida peer review statute and under the federal Health Care Quality Improvement Act and dismissed the case. Dr. Fullerton appealed only against the FMA. The Florida Court of Appeals held that neither the federal Health Care Quality Improvement Act nor the state peer review immunity statute protected the FMA from Dr. Fullerton's action. The court reversed the trial court's dismissal based on immunity and remanded the case, holding only that there was no immunity for FMA; the court expressed no opinion regarding the sufficiency of the complaint to state a cause of action.

Interestingly, a federal trial court in Kansas facing the same issue around the same time came to a contrary decision in *Bundren v. Parriott* [33]. After Dr. Bundren had provided expert testimony against Dr. Parriott in a medical malpractice case, Dr. Parriott complained about Dr. Bundren's testimony to the American College of Obstetricians and Gynecologists (ACOG). On the complaint form, Dr. Parriott answered "yes" to the question "Does this complaint involve a factual misrepresentation and/or perjury on fact-based issues as part of an expert witness' testimony?" Dr. Bundren (the expert) then sued Dr. Parriott (the doctor who filed the ACOG complaint) for defamation and malicious accusation of perjury based on the complaint form. Unlike the Florida court in the Fullerton case, this court held, among other things, that the ACOG complaint filed by Parriott is a "professional review action" that falls within the federal Health Care Quality Improvement Act, so there was immunity. This case was appealed and the Court of Appeals, in its unpublished opinion, affirmed the summary judgment for Dr. Parriott (who complained to ACOG) without addressing the Health Care Quality Improvement Act. The court found that Dr. Bundren failed to show that Dr. Parriott made defamatory statements, and that Dr. Parriott did not accuse Dr. Bundren of perjury merely by circling "yes" to question saying "factual misrepresentation and/or perjury."

Finally, in *Yancey v. Weis* [34], an ophthalmologist provided expert witness testimony for the plaintiff in a medical malpractice case; plaintiff won the case. Before the hearing on damages in the case, the expert received notice of an investigation by the American Academy of Ophthalmology (AAO). The complaint was filed by two AAO members (the defendant in the underlying medical malpractice case and the defendant's expert) asserting that the expert's testimony was misleading. The expert then sued AAO and the two physicians alleging defamation. The trial court dismissed the claim against the professional society holding that the expert, as a member of the AAO, agreed to abide by the AAO's ethical rules and regulations, which include peer review for questionable medical testimony. However, the court allowed the expert to proceed with suit against the two physicians individually for defamation when they filed their complaint with AAO.

13.3.5   Liability Points—Providing Expert Testimony

1. Immunity is not an absolute bar to liability.
2. Criminal prosecution, although rare, can happen.
3. State medical boards are increasing their regulation of testimony.
4. Professional organizations are engaging in more peer review of and discipline for expert testimony.

13.3.6   Risk Management Advice—Providing Expert Testimony

1. Understand the positions and expectations of:
    (a) State licensing boards—for your state and the state where testimony will be provided, if different;
    (b) Medical associations—AMA, state medical associations;
    (c) Specialty societies—APA, AAPL, etc.

2. Prepare adequately for the case—review all materials thoroughly.
3. Address weaknesses in the case with the retaining attorney.
4. Be able to effectively explain complex medicine to lay people.
5. Do not agree to be a patient's expert—avoid dual roles.

References

1. *Smith v. Welch*, 967 P.2d 727, 735 (Kan. 1998).
2. *Stanley v. McCarver*, 92 P.3d 849, 851-56 (Ariz. 2004).
3. *Martinez v. Lewis*, 969 P.2d 213, 218 n.4 (Colo. 1998).
4. *Harris v. Kreutzer*, 624 SE.2d 24, 27 (Va. 2006).
5. *Dyer v. Trachtman*, 679 NW.2d 311, 314-15 (Mich. 2004).
6. *Lambley v. Kameny*, 682 NE.2d 907 (Mass. App. Ct. 1997).
7. *Reed v. Bojarski*, 764 A.2d 433 (N.J. 2001).
8. *Pettus v. Cole*, 57 Cal. Rptr. 2d 46 (1996).
9. US Department of Health and Human Services, Regulation 45 CFR § 164.508(b)(4)(iii).
10. Office for Civil Rights, HIPAA Privacy Rule Enforcement Case Examples, at: http://www.hhs.gov/ocr/privacy/enforcement/examples/index..html (accessed February 17, 2010).
11. *Awai v. Kotin*, 872 P.2d 1332, 1336 (Colo. Ct. App. 1994).
12. *Parker v. Dodgion*, 971 P.2d 496, 498-99 (Utah 1998).
13. *Politi v. Tyler*, 751 A.2d 788, 791-92 (Vt. 2000).
14. *Dalton v. Miller*, 984 P.2d 666 (Colo. Ct. App. 2000).
15. Legal Opinions of the Attorney General of California, at: http://ag.ca.gov/opinions/pdfs/03-1201.pdf (accessed February 17, 2010).
16. *MacGregor v. Rutberg*, 478 F.3d 790 (7th Cir. 2007).
17. *Wilson v. Bernet*, 625 SE.2d 706, 714 (W.Va. 2005).
18. *LLMD of Mich., Inc. v. Jackson-Cross Co.*, 740 A.2d 186 (Pa. 1999) (involving a professional malpractice action against company for negligence in providing services as plaintiff's expert on issue of lost profits in federal lawsuit).
19. *Lambert v. Carneghi*, 70 Cal. Rptr. 3d 626 (Cal. Ct. App. 2008) (negligence claim against appraiser for failure to adequately define the correct standard and replacement cost of home destroyed by fire).
20. *Marrogi v. Howard*, 805 So.2d 1118, 1128 (La. 2002).
21. *Pace v. Swerdlow*, 519 F.3d 1067, 1069-70 (10th Cir. 2008).
22. *Levine v. Wiss & Co.*, 478 A.2d 397, 402 (N.J. 1984).
23. *Kobrin v. Gastfriend*, 821 NE.2d 60, 65 (Mass. 2005).
24. *Kutilek v. Gannon*, 766 F.Supp. 967, 973 (D. Kan. 1991).
25. Murphy, S.J., US Attorney, Eastern District of Michigan (2006). Press release "Miami Surgeon Indicted," December 1.
26. Murphy, S.J. , US Attorney, Eastern District of Michigan (2007). Press release "Miami Surgeon Pleads Guilty," September 20.
27. *Joseph v. D.C. Bd. of Med.*, 587 A.2d 1085 (D.C. Ct. App. 1991).
28. *In re Lustgarten*, 629 SE.2d 886, 892 (N.C. Ct. App. 2006).
29. APA (1996) Peer Review of Expert Testimony (Resource Document), APA Document Reference No. 960007.
30. AMA Policy Compendium (1998) Peer Review of Medical Expert Witness Testimony (Policy H-265.993).

31. *Austin v. Am. Ass'n of Neurological Surgeons*, 253 F.3d 967 (7th Cir. 2001), *cert. denied* 534 U.S. 1078 (2002).
32. *Fullerton v. FL Med. Ass'n, Inc.*, 938 So.2d 587 (Fla. Dist. Ct. App. 2006).
33. *Bundren v. Parriott*, 245 F. App'x 822 (10th Cir. 2007).
34. *Yancey v. Weis*, No. 27-CV-07-15651 (Minn., Hennepin Co. Dist. Ct.)

Index